Coping with Lymphedema

D0000262

Coping with Lymphedema

Joan Swirsky, RN
Diane Sackett Nannery

AVERY
a member of Penguin Putnam Inc.

The information and advice in this book are based on the training, personal experiences, and research of the authors. The contents are current and accurate; however, the information presented is not intended to substitute for professional medical advice. The authors and the publisher urge you to consult with your physician or other qualified health-care providers prior to starting any new treatment, or if you have any questions regarding a medical condition. Because there is always some risk involved, the author and publisher cannot be responsible for any adverse effects or consequences resulting from the use of any of the suggestions, preparations, or procedures described in this book.

Cover design: Eric Macaluso
Editor: Amy C. Tecklenburg
Typesetter: Al Berotti and Elaine V. McCaw

The figure on page 10 is adapted from a medical illustration by Orthoflex, Inc.

Avery
a member of
Penguin Putnam Inc.
375 Hudson Street
New York, NY 10014
www.penguinputnam.com

Library of Congress Cataloging-in-Publication Data

Swirsky, Joan.
    Coping with lymphedema : a practical guide to understanding, treating, and living with lymphedema / Joan Swirsky, Diane Sackett Nannery.
        p. cm.
    Includes bibliographical references and index.
    ISBN 0-89529-856-2 (pbk.)
    1. Lymphedema—Popular works. I. Nannery, Diane Sackett.
II. Title.
RC646.3.S94 1998
616.4'2—dc21   98-12066
                                                            CIP

Copyright © 1998 by Joan Swirsky and Diane Sackett Nannery

All rights reserved. No part of this publication may be reproduced, stored in a retrieval system, or transmitted, in any form or by any means, electronic, mechanical, photocopying, recording, information storage system, or otherwise, without the prior written permission of the copyright owner, except for the inclusion of brief quotations in a review.

Printed in the United States of America

10 9

Contents

From Joan Swirsky
To my husband, Steve,
my eternal source of inspiration and love.

From Diane Sackett Nannery
To Mom, Dad, and Bill, and to my husband Ed,
who has been there every step of the way.
Mostly, I dedicate this book to the memory
of my brother Bobby; I hope that I'm even
a little bit of what he thought I was.

Finally, we dedicate this book to all those brave
women, men, and children who have struggled with
and continue to suffer from lymphedema,
in the hope that it will inspire greater awareness,
increased research, preventive strategies,
and, ultimately, a cure.

Acknowledgments

We thank the hundreds of people with lymphedema who have contacted us—by phone, letter, and fax—for reaching out for advice and support. It is because of the urgency and desperation of your questions, and the widespread unavailability of answers, that we have written this book.

Heartfelt thanks to Rudy Shur of Avery Publishing Group for his invaluable help and guidance and for believing in the importance of bringing the subject of lymphedema to the public.

Deepest gratitude to our talented and brilliant editor, Amy Tecklenburg, who provided us with invaluable advice and guidance, many original ideas, and endless encouragement.

Great appreciation to Elana Hayden for her tireless research, astute suggestions, incredible Internet and World Wide Web expertise, and always-good-natured assistance.

Thank you to Ann Fonfa, a true student of lymphedema and crusader for those who suffer from this condition, for her generosity, time, and invaluable information.

Thank you to Diana Rulon, a pioneer in support and education of those affected by lymphedema.

Our gratitude to the dozens and dozens of dedicated lymphedema therapists we've spoken to across the country who greeted the advent of this book with warmth, encouragement, and enthusiasm. And special mention to those who helped us with invaluable information: Dana Wyrick, Arlette J. Dinclaux, Cheryl Morgan, Ph.D., Patricia Wiltse, and Kathie Cutler.

Also, our gratitude to Wendy Chaite for her time and effort in sharing with us crucial information about the new research being done on the genetic roots of primary lymphedema.

We thank Lori Kanestrin, OD and clinical nutritionist; Wesley B. Reiss, OD; and Carolyn Chambers Clark, EdD, RN, ARNP, FAAN, an alternative health practitioner, for their helpful information.

Special thanks to Dawn Mark-Lerner, a courageous young woman of 34 who contracted breast cancer just two years after she was married and who used her investigative skills to research all her options and decide against lymph-node removal. Dawn shared her research with us, steering us to those doctors who are studying ways to make nodal dissection and, by association, lymphedema, less widespread.

To Thomas R. Suozzi, Mayor and Supervisor of the City of Glen Cove, Long Island, our appreciation for being the perfect example of government in action by being the first regional elected official in the United States to act upon the fact that lymphedema is the kind of serious medical issue that demands and requires hospital and medical accountability.

To New York State Senator Kemp Hannon, our deep thanks for spearheading the pink-wristband policy in the New York State legislature.

To Doreen Banks, Town Councilwoman and health advocate from Long Island, New York, our thanks for bringing the issue of lymphedema before the wider public.

To Robert M. Kradjian, MD, and Christine Kradjian, a thank-you for your help in explaining the limitations of lymph-node removal and for your conviction that breast cancer can indeed be conquered.

To Rene Khafif, MD, we thank you for your generosity, time, and input, and for conducting the kind of cutting-edge research that ultimately may spare untold numbers of people the agonies of lymphedema.

To Deborah Sarnoff, MD, our sincere thanks for providing us with indispensable information about the dermatological aspects of lymphedema.

To Robert Lerner, MD, our appreciation for your pioneering efforts in establishing the first lymphedema center in the United States, and for sharing a wealth of information with us.

To Marvin Boris, MD, and Bonnie Lasinski, PT, our thanks for giving us an inside look at what a comprehensive lymphedema center should be, and for your helpful information.

To Judith Casley-Smith, PhD, and the late John Casley-Smith, MD, our appreciation for speaking to us from Australia and sharing the wealth of information you have acquired in your years of researching and treating lymphedema. To Maureen McDermott, loving thanks for her invaluable help in double-checking our resources.

Finally, our acknowledgment to Saskia Thiadens for the trailblazing work she has done for lymphedema patients and their therapists and doctors. Saskia singlehandedly founded the National Lymphedema Network and thus placed lymphedema "on the map" of public consciousness, where it belongs.

Preface

As a health and science journalist specializing in women's health issues, I have met, spoken to, and learned more than I dreamed there was to know about the lives of, women with breast cancer. Everything I learned infuriated me! As a woman, clinical nurse specialist, and resident of Long Island, New York—the "breast-cancer capital of the world"—I found what I learned about this widespread disease mystifying.

When I became an advocacy journalist for a regional newspaper, *The Women's Record*, and for other local newspapers, I addressed the powers that be in the political and scientific communities, challenging the questionable design of the Long Island Breast Cancer Study and investigating the possible links between breast cancer and the many environmental toxins and hazards that existed in our own and other areas.

For these publications, and for the Long Island section of *The New York Times*, I wrote about the political, environmental, sociological, psychological, and clinical aspects of this deadly disease. I even wrote a book about it. But in all of my writing, including my book—in which my coauthor and I included a chapter about the subject—I never appreciated the gravity or widespread nature of lymphedema.

It was not until Lorraine Pace from West Islip, Long Island—the first woman in the United States to map her own community's high incidence of breast cancer—introduced me to Diane Sackett Nannery that I fully comprehended lymphedema, yet another long-neglected aspect of the horrifying disease of breast cancer, as well as of many other conditions.

After inviting Diane to write an article for *REVOLUTION—The Journal of Nurse Empowerment*, the national publication of which I was then editor in chief, I became aware of the full implications of this lifelong condition and the degree to which it is unknown, not only to most breast-cancer patients, but to the many other people who are at risk of getting lymphedema, either as a result of undergoing lymph-node removal or for unknown reasons.

When I read Diane's article, I gained a deeper appreciation of the degree to which literally millions of people—men, women, and children—were suffering from lymphedema and had nowhere to go and no one to turn to for information. Within minutes of meeting each other, Diane and I determined to tell the world what lymphedema was all about.

We see this book as a kind of navigational guide for the journey of lymphedema. Both Diane and I want to put lymphedema on the map of the public's consciousness—to inspire greater awareness of this condition among both the lay public and medical practitioners. Hopefully, that awareness will lead to better research, greater prevention, and enhanced treatment.

Joan Swirsky

*   *   *   *

October is Breast-Cancer Awareness Month. It certainly was for me!

At 5:30 P.M. on October 1, my phone rang. As soon as I heard the doctor's voice, I knew there was a problem. After all, doctors don't usually call their patients unless the news is bad.

"The cells came back suspicious," he said. "I think our suspicions are correct."

"What suspicions?!" I wanted to scream. Five months before, I had been told that the lump in my left breast was nothing. Both my family doctor and my radiologist had assured me there had been no changes from my baseline mammogram.

But there I was, a woman who had done everything by the book—regular checkups, including breast exams, starting when I was twenty; monthly breast self-examinations beginning at twenty nine; and, following the American Cancer Society's recommendations, the baseline mammogram at the age of forty—a year before my breast-cancer diagnosis.

How did this happen? I thought that running to my doctor the moment I felt a lump in my breast would offer me at least the good prognosis many women are told early detection promises—if, in fact, breast cancer was the diagnosis. I thought my horrifying experience was unusual. But it wasn't! There are far too many stories like mine.

Yet maybe I was lucky. Because what I learned—early on—was that I had to take control, learn everything possible about my disease, and police each and every step of my treatment and recovery. Although I was just one of many patients my doctors had, I was the only me that I had, and I planned on being around for a long time.

My research came in handy when, immediately after my lumpectomy and axillary lymph-node dissection (removal of lymph nodes from the underarm area for examination), the nurses and aides attempted to take blood-pressure readings and blood samples from my left arm. I had read of the increased risk of infection and the possibility that the arm could develop lymphedema, so I requested not only that they use my right arm, but that they put up a sign over my bed alerting other members of the health-care team to leave my left arm alone.

Yet even this didn't work. The evening shift took my vital signs while I was half asleep, using only the light from the hall as illumination. They never even saw my sign! I kept asking myself, What about the women who don't even know about lymphedema or who may be too sedated to know what is being done to them?

Two days later, I returned home. Within minutes, I called my hospital to suggest they use a pink wristband to identify the affected arm of every breast-cancer patient who had undergone axillary node dissection. In the next few weeks, I wrote letters to seventy hospitals across the country and to every national breast-cancer and women's health organization I knew of.

Nursing magazines printed my letter and a national nursing magazine published an article I wrote about the pink wristband. The response was overwhelming—and continues to this day. It seemed that I had thought of a "better mousetrap," something hospitals and individual patients could use with little expense and great preventive potential.

Prior to my surgery, I had debated whether or not to have some of my axillary nodes removed. Unlike many of the women I spoke with (and have spoken to since), I knew the procedure would place restrictions on the affected arm for the rest of my life. An added concern was that the nodes were to be removed from my left underarm, and I am a lefty.

I read everything I could get my hands on about lymphedema. It wasn't enough to fill a pamphlet! But I was reassured by several best-selling books on breast cancer that lymphedema occurred in only about 5 percent of patients, and several doctors assured me that it was a condition seen primarily in patients who had had simple or radical mastectomies (complete removal of the breast).

Okay, I thought. I'm having a lumpectomy (removal of only the tumor and a bit of surrounding tissue), and I know what to do to avoid lymphedema. What I didn't know was that, like women all over the country, I wasn't being told the truth. Some so-called experts have even proclaimed publicly that doctors generally don't mention the possibility of getting lymphedema after breast-cancer surgery or radiation because they want to protect their patients from unnecessary anxiety. When a friend of mine—her arm horribly swollen from long neglect and a lack of medical attention—was told this by her own doctor, she blurted out to him, "You're going to 'protect' me into the grave!"

Nine months after my surgery, and two months after my follow-up chemotherapy and radiation treatments were over, I did develop lymphedema. It was only because of the research I had done that I knew what to do to keep it under control.

When I began my breast-cancer journey, I was a woman with questions. However, when it came to axillary node dissection and lymphedema, there were no answers. Through my research, I discovered the hidden, neglected side of lymphedema, a condition that counts among its victims thousands upon thousands of women and men who have survived surgery, radiation, and chemotherapy only to be faced with a permanent reminder of their disease—a reminder they were never warned about or taught how to manage. Throughout my experience, I kept wondering why no one had written a book about this. Then I met Joan Swirsky. Together we decided to write that book.

My interest in bringing this information to other people runs deep. For those who, like me, suffer from lymphedema, I want to validate its existence. I want to bring to public attention the impact it has on our lives. It is also my hope, and Joan's, that this information will prompt research funding, treatment options, and—dare we hope it?—a cure!

Diane Sackett Nannery

Part I

Lymphedema: An Overview

Introduction

When she was 47, Catherine had a lumpectomy for breast cancer, during which several of her lymph nodes were removed to check for the cancer's spread. Her surgery was followed by six weeks of radiation therapy. "Then I got back to my old self," she said.

A few months later, she woke up one morning to find her arm and hand hugely swollen. She went immediately to her doctor, who told her the swelling was normal after such surgery and she might find relief by elevating her arm. But elevation didn't help, and Catherine spent the next two years suffering with her swollen limb. Then she read a small article in *Coping* magazine about lymphedema.

"If I had known I was vulnerable to this condition and that there was help for it," she said, "those two years of agony might have been avoided. Now I tell everyone about it; if I save one person from the distress I had, it's worth it."

As Catherine learned the hard way, it is largely up to the individual to educate him- or herself about lymphedema's risks, to inform others who may be suffering from the condition or at risk of developing it, and to bring this information to doctors, lymphedema therapists, and any other people who may be involved in his or her treatment, including insurance companies.

It is not only cancer survivors who must become aware of this condition. Anyone whose lymphatic system has been damaged, whether through accident, surgery, or any other means, is vulnerable. Some people develop lymphedema unrelated to any other known condition. Even infants and children may be stricken with lymphedema.

In Part I, we will answer many of the questions the condition raises, describing what lymphedema is, the many problems that invariably go along with it, how it is diagnosed, who is at risk for it, and what those who are at risk can do to reduce their chances of developing it.

1
What Is Lymphedema?

Lymphedema is a combination of two words: *lymph* (a natural body fluid) and *edema* (swelling)—literally, it means "swelling caused by lymph." This is a chronic disorder in which lymph fails to circulate properly and, as a result, accumulates in the tissues of a limb or other part of the body. Its symptoms can include pain, numbness, a loss of mobility, a loss of skin elasticity, hardening of the skin, increased susceptibility to infection, chronic ulceration of the skin, and swelling that can make an arm, leg, or other body part as much as two, three, four, or even more times its normal size. Once the onset of lymphedema takes place, it affects every facet of your life—and it never goes away. If untreated, the damage it causes is irreversible and progressive.

In order to understand this condition, it is first necessary to understand how the body's circulatory systems work, and also to understand the role of the immune system. As you will see, these systems are separate, yet intrinsically related.

THE BODY'S CIRCULATORY SYSTEMS

When we think of circulation, we tend to think of blood and the blood vessels. But the body has another circulatory system that works in concert with the blood system. This is the lymphatic system. The lymphatic system is a mechanism for removing excess blood protein and water from the spaces around the cells and returning them to the blood system.

The Blood System

Blood is composed of red blood cells, which carry oxygen; white blood cells, which fight infection; platelets, which stop bleeding; and

5

plasma, the liquid portion, which is 90 percent water and also contains a number of proteins that are essential to life. Blood is pumped through the blood vessels by the heart. Upon leaving the heart, the blood goes first to the lungs, where it picks up oxygen. It then travels to the cells of the body by means of the arteries and capillaries. Since capillaries are somewhat porous, they allow for oxygen and nutrients to be transferred out of the blood by means of the plasma and to enter the tissues, where they are used to produce the energy needed to carry out all the activities necessary for life.

When fluid diffuses out of the capillaries, it joins the interstitial fluid, which is found in spaces between the body's cells and tissues. It is the interstitial fluid that bathes all the cells of the body and serves as an exchange medium for the nutrients carried in the blood. From this fluid, oxygen and nutrients enter the cells. In turn, the cells release carbon dioxide and other cellular waste products and eliminate them through the circulatory system. The blood is returned to the heart by means of the veins and the journey begins all over again.

As blood passes through the capillaries in the tissues, there is a continual exchange of its plasma portion (the liquid and nutrients, including protein molecules, that are needed by the cells for the maintenance of life) and the interstitial fluid. Normally, the amount of fluid that exits the capillaries for the interstitial fluid is roughly equal to the amount of fluid that reenters the capillaries from the interstitial fluid. However, a small percentage of the fluid is left behind. It is this fluid that must rejoin the blood circulation by means of the lymphatic system.

The Lymphatic System

The lymphatic system consists of the lymph, lymphatic vessels, and lymph nodes. It is responsible for returning excess fluid and blood protein from the tissues to the blood circulation, and also plays an important role in protecting the body against illness.

Lymph is a clear, colorless fluid composed of water, protein, salts, glucose, and urea, plus white blood cells. Basically, lymph is interstitial fluid that has left the tissue spaces and entered the lymphatic capillaries. Unlike the blood vessels, which are closed (that is, the blood is always contained within the blood vessels), the lymphatic system's capillaries are open at one end. It is through these openings that the interstitial fluid enters the capillaries to become lymph. At the other end, lymphatic capillaries join with other lymphatic capillaries to form the lymphatic vessels.

These vessels act as channels through which lymph is moved through the body, back toward the blood circulation. The lymph is as thick as honey or syrup and it moves rather slowly, its movement powered by the contractions of skeletal muscles and the motion of breathing. An amazingly efficient system of one-way valves within the lymphatic vessels prevents the fluid from flowing backward toward the tissues again. Lymphatic vessels also absorb most of the digested fats that drain from the intestines, and transport these to the bloodstream as well. This intestinal lymphatic fluid is called chyle and often appears whitish because of its fat content.

As lymph is transported through the body, it passes through structures called lymph nodes, which are located along the lymphatic vessels in various regions of the body. These round or kidney-shaped nodes, roughly the size of lima beans, are found in the head and neck, armpits, groin, abdomen, pelvis, and chest, either deep in the body or near to the surface, where they can be detected through manual examination. There are between 500 and 1,500 lymph nodes in the body.

The lymph nodes have two main functions. First, they produce lymphocytes, which are white blood cells that combat infection by producing antibodies to fight bacteria and viruses. Second, they filter the lymph, destroying and removing dead cells and waste materials, as well as bacteria, viruses, and other potential disease-causing pathogens. In essence, the nodes catch and annihilate these toxins, preventing them from entering the bloodstream and wreaking havoc there. When the lymph nodes have performed their detoxifying function, the lymphatic fluid is ready to be returned to the blood.

At the end of the lymphatic system, the lymphatic vessels join together to form the two lymphatic ducts. The ducts connect the lymphatic circulation with the blood circulation; through them, lymphatic fluid passes back into the blood. The left duct, which is the larger of the two, serves as the drainage system for 80 percent of the body, including the left side of the neck and head, the left arm, the trunk of the body, and the legs. This duct begins in the area of the lower spine, collecting the lymph from all the lymphatic vessels of the lower limbs, pelvis, abdomen, and lower chest. The fluid is then transported up to the chest, where it empties into the central blood circulation through a vein at the base of the left side of the neck. The right lymphatic duct collects lymph from the right side of the neck,

Understanding Body Fluids

The main constituent in the human body is water, averaging approximately 60 percent of body weight for men and 55 percent for women. With age, the percentage decreases to approximately 45 to 55 percent in older adults. The fluids in the body contain solutes, which are dissolved solid substances known as electrolytes and nonelectrolytes. Electrolytes are mineral compounds that carry an electrical charge. These include sodium, potassium, chloride, and phosphate. Nonelectrolytes include glucose (simple sugar) and urea.

Throughout the body, fluids are found in two compartments: the intracellular (fluid found within cells) and the extracellular (fluid found outside of individual cells). Approximately two-thirds of the body's fluid is intracellular, while one-third is extracellular. The extracellular fluid includes plasma, the liquid portion of the blood; lymph; interstitial fluid, which surrounds and bathes the cells and is the source of lymphatic fluid; and transcellular fluid, specialized fluids that are separated from the interstitial fluid by membranes. The latter category includes cerebrospinal fluid (the fluid that bathes and cushions the brain and spinal cord), pericardial fluid (a thin layer of fluid that surrounds the heart), pleural fluid (a thin layer of fluid that surrounds the lungs), synovial fluid (fluid that lubricates the joints), intraocular fluids (fluids that bathe and nourish the eyes), and digestive secretions. The fluid compartments in the body are separated by permeable membranes that allow the movement of water and solutes. While water and some small molecules can move easily between compartments, proteins do not cross the membranes with ease.

Edema is the swelling of tissue due to an accumulation of fluid. Ordinary edema usually indicates an expansion of the volume of interstitial fluid, the result of obstruction in the veins, heart failure, inflammation, or increased retention of sodium and water. Its symptoms may include swelling of the ankles, legs, and/or fingers, or puffiness around the eyes. Treatment usually involves restriction of sodium and fluids, the use of support hose, diuretic therapy (water pills) to increase the excretion of sodium and water through the kidneys, and, in extreme cases, dialysis.

In contrast, the swelling caused by lymphedema arises when the lymphatic system—lymphatic vessels or lymph nodes or both—is damaged and cannot transport lymph back to the blood circulation.

When this happens, large protein and fat molecules collect in the interstitial spaces and chronic inflammation and scar tissue develop. Because its normal flow is impeded, lymphatic fluid backs up, causing the swelling called lymphedema. While restriction of sodium and fluids may help to reduce some of the swelling, diuretics are of limited value in treating lymphedema. In fact, the International Society of Lymphology Executive Committee reports that although diuretics may occasionally be useful during the initial phase of treatment, long-term use of these drugs is of marginal benefit and may cause complications such as electrolyte (body chemistry) disturbances. In addition, because diuretics move fluids out of the body so effectively, they may be dangerous to patients with certain cardiac conditions, deep venous thrombosis (blood clots in the veins), or congestive heart failure.

the right chest area, and the right arm, and empties into a vein in the right side of the neck.

CIRCULATION AND THE IMMUNE SYSTEM

As we have seen, the circulatory systems are central to nourishing the tissues, removing wastes, and maintaining the body's critical fluid balance. That is not their only role, however. They also are important components of the immune system.

The immune system is that complex mechanism that defends and protects the body against the bacterial and viral invaders that threaten to undermine our health and well-being. To be sure, our bodies have other ways of warding off infections and diseases. Among them are the skin, which covers and protects the entire body; the mucous membranes that line our breathing passages and snare or sweep away minute organisms; our temperature-regulating mechanism, which elevates body temperature to destroy organisms that cannot withstand the heat; and even our sticky earwax, salty tears, and acidic stomach juices, all of which protect against and can destroy or retard the growth of microorganisms.

But if these defenses fail to ward off bacterial or viral invasion, the body depends on its second line of defense: blood and lymph. At the first sign of foreign invasion, blood and lymph containing infection-fighting white blood cells rush to the affected tissues in an attempt to

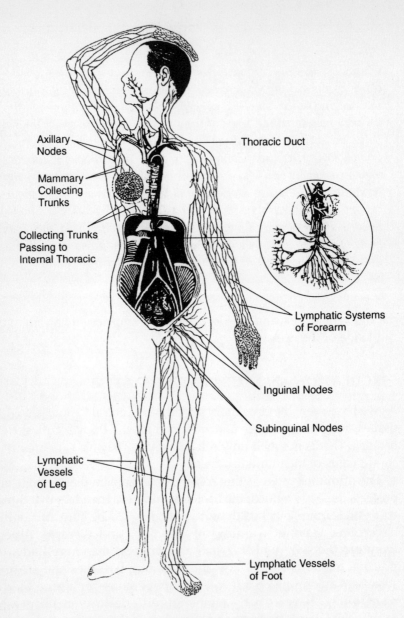

Axillary
Nodes

Mammary
Collecting
Trunks

Collecting Trunks
Passing to
Internal Thoracic

Thoracic Duct

Lymphatic Systems
of Forearm

Inguinal Nodes

Subinguinal Nodes

Lymphatic
Vessels
of Leg

Lymphatic Vessels
of Foot

Figure 1.1   The Lymphatic System

Lymphatic vessels and lymph nodes are found throughout the body, but
tend to be concentrated in certain areas. Note the numbers of lymphatic
vessels in the hands and breast area, for instance, and the concentration
of lymph nodes in the head and neck, armpits, and groin. Lymph rejoins
the blood circulation by means of the right lymphatic duct and the
thracic duct, located at the right and left sides of the neck, respectively.

localize the infection and prevent its spread. Different types of white blood cells perform different functions. Some physically attack, engulf, and consume invading organisms; others secrete substances that kill specific enemies. Once infection has been contained, the debris resulting from this cellular warfare is cleaned up by means of the lymphatic circulation—it enters the lymphatic capillaries with the interstitial fluid and is filtered out by the lymph nodes. The purified lymphatic fluid is then reintroduced into the blood system.

THE EFFECTS OF LYMPHATIC DAMAGE

If the lymphatic system is damaged, its normal functions are compromised. If the nodes are injured, they cannot filter toxins from the system or produce the lymphocytes that fight infection; if nodes are removed, this leaves the body with fewer nodes to fight disease and also disrupts the pathways by which lymph is normally drained from the tissues; if the vessels are injured, they can no longer transport lymph through the system as they should. Put simply, a damaged lymphatic system works inefficiently, giving rise to symptoms that demand treatment.

Both blood plasma and interstitial fluid contain protein, but plasma normally contains about 7 percent protein, whereas interstitial fluid contains approximately 2 percent. Biochemically, this results in most plasma protein being held in the circulatory system. If some leaks out, it is returned to the blood by the lymphatic circulation. However, if the lymphatic system is damaged, a concentration of protein eventually accumulates in the tissues. This protein further interferes with the flow of tissue fluid into the lymphatic capillaries and, ultimately, the blood. The result is edema, or swelling.

How might the lymphatic system be damaged? The filtering mechanism of the lymph nodes or the lymphatic vessels may be injured as a result of surgery, injury, infection, invading cancer cells, a congenital or acquired malformation or obstruction of the veins, or radiation treatment.[1] One common scenario that can lead to damage is cancer surgery. If there is cancer anywhere in the body, its cells may enter the draining lymphatic vessels and be carried to other parts of the body. So for the purpose of determining if cancer is present or has spread, lymph nodes are often removed for microscopic examination to determine whether they are cancerous or noncancerous.

Whatever the cause of the damage, a damaged lymphatic system is unable to tolerate the demand for the drainage of lymph fluid. In short order, large molecules of proteins and lipids (fats) accumulate in the interstitial spaces, surrounding tissues are deprived of their vital oxygen supply, and chronic inflammation and scar tissue develop, which further impedes the flow of lymph. The result: a backup of fluid and swelling in the affected limb—lymphedema. The trapped protein becomes stagnant, creating an environment ripe for infection. At the same time, because the lymphatic system is an important component of the immune system, the immune response is often impaired. The result can be repeated bouts of infectious disease.

Some doctors refer to lymphedema as a "plumbing problem." In fact, this analogy is quite apt. It is as if water were coming into your home through three underground pipes, but one of the pipes—the one with a filter to remove impurities—is damaged and has become clogged with dirt. It is easy to see why this would severely compromise both the purity and the flow of water, as well as resulting in a backup of water.

Your lymphatic vessels can be compared to the pipes in this illustration; your lymphatic fluid to the water; and the accumulating protein to the dirt. If the flow of lymph through lymphatic vessels is impeded, both by injury to the vessels and by the resulting accumulation of protein molecules, the backup that ensues is forced into the tissues of the affected arm or leg, creating a seriously swollen limb.

TYPES OF LYMPHEDEMA

There are two general categories of lymphedema, primary and secondary. Primary lymphedema is lymphedema unrelated to any other known condition. Secondary lymphedema is lymphedema acquired as a result of some other disease or trauma.

Approximately 1 in 6,000 people in the United States is affected by hereditary primary lymphedema. The symptoms of type I hereditary lymphedema, also known as Milroy's Disease, are typically present at birth, and the swelling tends to worsen slowly with advancing age. This type of lymphedema affects more females than males.

In type II hereditary lymphedema, or Meige disease, symptoms usually develop during childhood, adolescence, or early adulthood. This form of the disease generally produces severe swelling in areas below the waist, with the first symptoms usually including reddened skin over areas of swelling. This type of lymphedema affects males and females in equal numbers. Lymphedema tarda is a form of hereditary lymphedema that usually occurs after the age of thirty-five. Its symptoms are similar to those of type II hereditary lymphedema.

In the hereditary form of the disease, symptoms of lymphedema develop because the lymphatic vessels are obstructed as a result of malformation of the lymphatic system. In some cases, there may be fewer lymphatic vessels than normal or the vessels may be underdeveloped. In other cases, lymphatic vessels may be unusually large and numerous.

Complications of hereditary lymphedema may include lymphangitis (inflammation of lymphatic vessels) and cellulitis (these conditions will be discussed in detail in Chapter 2). Red streaks on the skin may develop, as may a general feeling of ill health, fever, chills, and/or headaches. Some people with this condition develop a persistent accumulation of fluid in the lungs. The most serious long-term complication of all forms of hereditary lymphedema is a slightly increased risk of developing lymphangiosarcoma, a type of cancer, in the affected area.

Most cases of congenital lymphedema are inherited as what geneticists call an autosomal dominant trait. Simply put, if an individual inherits a defective copy of a certain gene, from either the mother or the father, he or she will be affected. This is because the defective gene will "dominate" the corresponding normal gene received from the other parent, resulting in the appearance of the disease. If an affected person has children with an unaffected partner, the likelihood of any individual child inheriting a defective gene, and thus the disorder, is 50 percent, regardless of the sex of the child. It is also possible for congenital lymphedema to occur because of genetic mutation (a spontaneous change in genetic material) early in fetal development. Once such a mutation occurs, it can be passed down to the affected individual's offspring.

Secondary lymphedema is lymphedema that comes about as a result of illness or injury that damages the lymphatic system. It is much more common than primary lymphedema. It can occur after surgery with lymph-node removal, after radiation therapy, or after an injury to or infection of the lymphatic system. This is because these factors can result in lymphatic vessels being severed, damaged, or blocked. Sometimes kidney failure or heart problems may lead to lymphedema in one or both legs. In such cases it is likely to remain undiagnosed and be either ignored or treated improperly.

Primary and secondary lymphedema are equally threatening, and affect both children and adults.

SYMPTOMS OF LYMPHEDEMA

Lymphedema is a serious condition involving the lymphatic, circulatory, and immune systems, which cannot be seen with the naked eye. What can be seen, as a kind of bold representation of the inner damage that has taken place, are swelling of the limb and changes in the skin.

The first symptoms of lymphedema may be subtle, starting when you notice that the ring on your finger is hard to remove, or that your arm appears slightly swollen, or that you seem to have a minor infection from the scratch of a pin. Or they may be quite blatant—a sudden ballooning of an arm or leg or a lack of mobility in the affected limb.

Swelling

Lymphedema often begins with a condition called pitting edema, in which the tissues swell due to an excess of fluid and small indentations form when the affected area is pressed with a finger. In pitting edema, the indentations return to normal if the area is elevated, and no noticeable or lasting changes are apparent. This is considered grade one, or acute, lymphedema. Without careful monitoring and treatment, a person with acute lymphedema is at risk of progressing to grade two lymphedema, usually after three to six months.

In grade two lymphedema, the condition becomes chronic. As it does so—and especially if left untreated—it involves less pitting edema, but significant skin changes set in. The affected limb swells, but the swelling is not reduced by elevation. In addition, the skin hardens as fibrous tissue develops, and the skin does not pit when pressed. This hardened tissue further blocks the fluid's flow, which makes the lymphedema worse. It is at this point—when the thick, coarse skin may become ulcerated and bacteria are able to enter the skin—that a person becomes vulnerable to cellulitis, an infection of the soft tissues of the skin. Grade three lymphedema occurs after repeated attacks of cellulitis. If a lower limb is affected, it can lead to a chronic condition known as lymphostatic elephantiasis, in which the leg becomes hugely enlarged and the skin and underlying tissue become hardened. The term *elephantiasis* is used to describe the similarity in appearance to an elephant's leg.

Skin Changes and Problems

It is important to understand the role the skin plays in lymphedema, not only because it often reflects the severity of the disorder but because it is so visible to the outside world. Your appearance affects how you feel about yourself, and also affects your ability to proceed with a normal work and social life. According to Deborah Sarnoff, MD, a clinical professor in the Department of Dermatology at New York University Medical School who has treated the skin problems of many people with lymphedema, people suffer as much from the change in the appearance of their skin as they do from the discomfort and potential danger of the other symptoms of this stubborn condition. It is therefore crucial to treat skin problems before they reach an advanced stage.

When lymphatic vessels are obstructed or destroyed, they are unable to drain away microbes that can colonize in the tissues and penetrate the skin. In short order, this protein-rich, stagnant lymph creates a perfect environment for bacteria to grow and flourish, leading to chronic dermatitis (skin inflammation), hyperkeratosis (patches of roughened skin), and a brawny or leathery appearance. The skin may also become warty or horny or callused. In addition, there may be significant disfigurement, with the limb swelling to several times its normal size. Often, there is weeping of lymphatic fluid through the skin, giving the skin a mossy texture. Chronic weeping, leaking, and oozing leads to a mushy softening of the skin that can give rise to additional bacterial, yeast, and/or fungal infections—a kind of vicious cycle.

For example, a fungal infection such as athlete's foot may develop in the spaces between the toes, causing peeling and scaling and a breakdown of the skin. Once an opening in the skin occurs, a portal for infectious organisms exists. *Staphylococcus* or *Streptococcus* bacteria may enter the system, thrive in the stagnant lymphatic fluid, and cause repeated bouts of infection. As this vicious cycle continues, the individual may experience a loss of normal sensation, a lack of mobility, and a diminishing sense of self-esteem as a result of the limb's unsightly appearance.

Once lymphedema becomes chronic, changes occur in the dermis, which is the deeper layer of skin. In addition to swelling of the lymphatic vessels, there is a thickening of the skin and a development of scarlike formations called fibrosis. Since early diagnosis of both skin and other problems is the key to better overall health, and in some cases longer survival, all patients with chronic lymphedema must undergo regular skin examinations on a lifelong basis.

Very rarely, lymphangiosarcoma, a form of cancer that affects the tissues of the lymphatic system, may develop as a complication of chronic lymphedema. The reason or reasons for this are not well understood, but it may be related to the degeneration of collagen (a protein that is a key component of skin tissues) and fats below the dermis, or to impairment of the immune system in people with lymphedema.[2] Anyone with lymphedema who suddenly develops crops of purple-red patches or bumps on the skin of the involved limb should consult a doctor without hesitation, as these are the primary symptoms of lymphangiosarcoma. If a doctor suspects lymphangiosarcoma, a biopsy should be performed at once.

DIAGNOSING LYMPHEDEMA

Often, people with symptoms of lymphedema hesitate to seek help, either because they think those symptoms will go away, or because they believe the symptoms "go along with" their cancer surgery or accident. However, since diagnosis is the first step toward treatment and effective management, any person who has had a traumatic accident, undergone surgery in which lymph nodes were removed, or been through any kind of radiation treatment must pay close attention to any signs of swelling and seek medical advice immediately.

When you go to your doctor, you may find that he or she knows about as much—or as little—about the condition as you do. There are no standard criteria for diagnosing lymphedema. One doctor may depend on visual examination, another on imaging scans, yet another on arm or leg measurements that chart the course of swelling. Some doctors combine these methods to arrive at a definitive diagnosis. Many people actually end up diagnosing themselves.

However it is done, getting a correct diagnosis is essential if you are to proceed with effective treatment—treatment that will manage the condition before it gets worse.

Measuring

One way to assess lymphedema is to measure the affected limb. Using an ordinary tape measure, your doctor measures the circumference of your limb in several places to monitor the increase or decrease in swelling on an ongoing basis. In an arm, measurements are taken in at least one location on the lower arm and two locations on the upper arm; this may be reversed for a leg. It is important that both the affected limb and its unaffected counterpart be measured.

Having one limb somewhat larger than the other does not necessarily mean there is anything wrong. If you are right-handed, for instance, your right arm may naturally be a little larger than your left. In fact, a healthy dominant arm may even be larger than a swollen nondominant arm. Generally, however, if one limb is two centimeters (about three-quarters of an inch) larger than the other, a doctor may make a diagnosis of lymphedema. Even with such a relatively small degree of swelling, you are likely to experience a feeling of heaviness or fullness in the affected limb. A difference of two and a half centimeters (about one inch) indicates moderate lymphedema.

Another way of measuring the limb is to submerge it in water and measure the volume of displaced liquid. But even though this method is highly accurate, it is rarely used because of its messy nature.

Imaging

In addition to measuring your limbs, your physician may recommend that you see a radiologist, a medical doctor who specializes in the use and interpretation of x-ray tests for diagnosis and treatment. This professional may perform one or more different tests to visualize the condition of the lymphatic system and to determine where any blockages may be. These tests include the color flow Doppler, magnetic resonance imaging (MRI), lymphangioscintigraphy (LAS), and a computerized tomography (CT) scan.

Color Flow Doppler

Through the use of ultrasound technology, this noninvasive technique creates an image of the flow of fluids through the vascular system and detects any blockages. To perform this test, the doctor places blood-pressure cuffs on different areas of the limb to measure the highest blood pressure of the artery. Then the cuffs are attached to a machine that measures the amplitude of the sound at each cuff. The test takes approximately fifteen minutes to perform.

Magnetic Resonance Imaging (MRI)

This test detects abnormalities of the circulatory system, discriminating between the muscle, fat, and fluid, as well as determining the extent of underlying tissue damage. It also shows enlarged lymph nodes, but not tumors or obstructions.

To undergo this test, you lie in a tunnel-shaped electromagnetic machine that is open at both ends. Short bursts of alternating electromagnetic energy—not radiation—emit tiny signals that are used to create cross-sectioned images of the area being observed.

While the process is lengthy—it takes about an hour—and requires you to remain immobile, it causes no discomfort or pain. However, according to a study published in the *Journal of the American Medical Association*, nearly 30 percent of those who undergo this test suffer anxiety-related reactions in the confinement of the machine. Some radiologic centers now have "open" MRI machines for people who tend to experience claustrophobia. The new machine has open ends and sides, allowing you a full range of movement of your limbs and an unobstructed view in four different directions.

Lymphangioscintigraphy (LAS)

This is an invasive test in which a radioactive solution is injected into the tissues. Images are obtained as the radiotracer travels through the lymphatic system, creating detailed pictures of lymphatic channels and lymph nodes.

A combination of MRI and LAS is considered highly effective in viewing the lymphatic system, since MRI alone cannot detect abnormalities or other problems in the veins or arteries. MRI gives important information about soft tissues, lymph nodes, and blood vessels, and is particularly useful for determining whether vessels are obstructed, while LAS depicts the lymphatic channels and the functioning of the lymphatic system.

Computerized Tomography (CT)

This technology is sometimes used to help diagnose lymphedema. However, it involves doses of radiation and sometimes the injection of a contrast dye into the veins, which has the potential to cause severe allergic reactions. Therefore, many doctors prefer MRI scans. There are also other tests, such as venography and lymphography, that can be used to assess the functioning of the circulatory systems. However, these tests too involve injecting dyes into the veins, and they are associated with a high incidence of complications, including permanent swelling. As a result, these tests are not among the first choices for diagnosing lymphedema.

In spite of the seriousness and widespread incidence of lymphedema, few people have ever heard of it. It has been hidden from view by those who suffer in silence with its symptoms; by a medical system that offers a cornucopia of treatments for all sorts of other ailments but no comprehensive preventive or treatment strategies for lymphedema; and by a scientific community that has few research projects designed to give us a better understanding of how to prevent or treat this lifelong condition.

Thousands of people each year become vulnerable to lymphedema. Many of them might be able to avoid the condition altogether—if they learn what makes them vulnerable and what strategies might be employed to prevent it or, if necessary, to manage the condition once it appears. We will explore these subjects in the chapter that follows.

2
Who Is Vulnerable to Lymphedema?

Cancer. Accident. Birth defect. These are words that strike fear into every person's heart. Yet we now live in a world in which more people are living with cancer than are dying from it. More people are benefiting from advances in trauma medicine and surviving accidents. And increasing numbers of birth defects are being diagnosed early and treated effectively.

So grateful are the recipients of life-saving surgery and treatment that they often accept the side effects of treatment—no matter how difficult—as something they have to learn to live with. And often, that's true. After chemotherapy or radiation therapy, many people feel less energetic than they did before treatment. Surgery may leave a person using a cane or wheelchair or getting used to a prosthesis. Birth defects often carry with them the need for lifelong adjustments and ongoing care.

But most people who have lymphedema never had any idea they were at risk for the condition or why. They merely arose one day to find an arm or leg swollen beyond recognition. In some cases—in primary lymphedema, for example—it is not known what leads to the condition. In other cases, however, we can point to certain events that we know put people at risk. These include treatment for cancer, especially breast cancer; trauma; and infection.

BREAST CANCER

Each year, more than 182,000 American women are diagnosed with breast cancer. Approximately 89 percent of them undergo surgery involving removal of underarm lymph nodes. In the United States, the majority of women are eligible for breast-conserving surgical treatment (better known as lumpectomy), and almost every woman who opts for this surgery undergoes lymph-node removal. Thus, approximately 161,000 women with breast cancer undergo lymph-node removal each year. Of these, an estimated 35 to 40 percent develop some degree of lymphedema. Experts calculate that if a woman has eight to ten lymph nodes removed, her risk of developing lymphedema is 50 percent. If she has twenty or more lymph nodes removed, the risk rises sharply.[1] Lymphedema is unpredictable, however. Some people who have comparatively few lymph nodes removed develop the condition while others who have numerous nodes removed never get lymphedema. Further, there is no telling when the condition might occur since it may appear months, even years, after the lymphatic system has been compromised. All in all, it has been estimated that over 3 million American women who currently have breast cancer will develop some degree of lymphedema.[2]

Until relatively recently, most doctors believed that only women who had mastectomies were at risk, particularly those who underwent the procedure known as the Halsted radical mastectomy. This type of surgery was introduced in the late nineteenth century by Dr. William Halsted, and it continued to be standard operating procedure for breast cancer until the 1960s. In the Halsted radical mastectomy, the affected breast, the chest muscle beneath it, and all of the lymph nodes under the arm on that side are removed.

Today, the Halsted procedure is virtually extinct, replaced by the modified radical mastectomy (in which only the breast and a sampling of lymph nodes are removed) and, increasingly, lumpectomy (in which only the lump and a small area of surrounding tissue are removed).[3] The number of lymph nodes removed in these procedures varies. First, the number of nodes under any person's arms may range from a few to up to 150 or even more. Second, doctors differ in their standard practice. Some remove only three nodes for microscopic examination; others remove thirty or more.

Despite the less extreme nature of current surgical techniques, greater numbers of women are getting lymphedema. This may be because radiation treatments routinely follow lumpectomy, and radiation may be absorbed by and thus destroy lymphatic tissue.[4] Radiation can damage lymph nodes by causing the formation of scar tissue, and it can increase the scarring or destruction of the lymphatic vessels. Several studies have found that women who had radiation treatment directed at the area from which lymph nodes were removed were significantly more likely to develop lymphedema.[5]

Anyone who has lymph nodes removed is vulnerable to lym-

Rethinking Lymph-Node Removal

Lymph-node removal is a major risk factor for lymphedema. Today, lymph nodes are removed for two reasons: to see if they are cancerous and, if cancer is diagnosed, to do what the medical profession refers to as staging. *Staging allows doctors to understand how advanced the cancer is, which in turn aids in planning further treatment, such as radiation, chemotherapy, or hormonal therapy. Typically, three to fifteen nodes are removed for these purposes, although some doctors routinely remove up to thirty.*

It is important to note that doctors have to remove lymph nodes to see if, in fact, disease is present in them. While they may have a "clinical impression" that the nodes are diseased, they don't know this until the nodes are examined microscopically by a pathologist. Lymph nodes are removed in most operations for cases of suspected invasive (rather than in situ, *or confined) cancer.*

Yet not all experts agree on the necessity of removing lymph nodes routinely. Robert M. Kradjian, MD, a breast surgeon and author of Save Your Life From Breast Cancer *(Berkley, 1994), believes that underarm lymph-node removal (known to surgeons as* axillary dissection) *is not necessary in every case of breast cancer.[1] Clinical trials, Dr. Kradjian says, demonstrate no difference in survival rates between breast-cancer patients who have undergone lymph-node removal and those who have not. Dr. Kradjian points to several circumstances under which he believes breast-cancer patients would be wise (or at least justified) in electing* not *to have lymph nodes removed:*

• *If chemotherapy will be administered. This is most likely to apply to younger patients, since chemotherapy has been shown to have definite benefits for premenopausal women with breast cancer, but it is not as effective for postmenopausal women. Moreover, many doctors recommend against chemotherapy for people over the age of sixty-five because its side effects may be too damaging.*

• *If the patient is elderly.*

• *If the patient chooses not to have chemotherapy.*

• *If the tumor is five centimeters (about two and a half inches) in diameter or less. (Anything over five centimeters is considered a large tumor.)*

• *If there is no indication that removing the lymph nodes will improve the patient's prognosis—for example, if the cancer has spread widely throughout the body and this has been established by other tests, such as lung scans, bone scans, and blood tests.*

Some practitioners question the very practice of staging. Richard G. Margolese, MD, a professor of surgical oncology at McGill University in Montreal, believes that the use of this method to determine the risk of recurrence of breast cancer is based on a concept that is probably incorrect, and that identifying those individuals who are most likely to benefit from chemotherapy is more important than identifying those whose cancer had spread.[2] In fact, he says, if all breast-cancer patients were given chemotherapy, there would be no need for lymph-node dissection at all. Peter J. Deckers, MD, chair of the Department of Surgery at the University of Connecticut School of Medicine, goes even further. He cites a clinical trial of the National Institutes of Health's National Surgical Adjuvant Breast and Bowel Project (NSABP) that found no advantage (in terms of survival) to undergoing lymph-node removal, and he predicts that the practice of lymph-node dissection will be extinct within the next decade.[3]

Other researchers are experimenting with alternative approaches to lymph-node removal. Dr. David Krag, a breast surgeon and associate professor in general surgery at the University of Vermont, pioneered a technique in which a minute amount of radioactive tracer is injected into the perimeter of a breast tumor immediately before surgery. Then a highly sensitive and precise probe is used to detect the radioactive material as it reaches the lymphatic system. The first lymph gland it reaches is the one that is actually draining that particular tumor. Once located, that single gland—which researchers have named the "sentinel lymph node"—is removed, tagged as the sentinel gland, and examined microscopically. In Dr. Krag's original sentinel-node experiment with fifty-five patients, examination of the sentinel node accurately predicted whether cancer had spread to other lymph nodes in 100 percent of cases.

If these results can be duplicated with a larger number of cases, researchers believe it will prove that it is unnecessary to remove lymph glands from patients whose sentinel lymph nodes show no sign of cancer. Based on Dr. Krag's work, Rene Khafif, MD, Director of Surgical Oncology at Maimonides Medical Center in Brooklyn, New York, is conducting research with his colleagues and with scientists from fifteen other major medical centers throughout the United States on a minimal surgical procedure done under local anesthesia that attempts to identify the specific individuals whose cancer has spread into the lymph nodes.[4] The ultimate goal of this research is to learn if the findings in the sentinel node can accurately predict whether or not the other glands are affected by the cancer, and thus to eliminate the need to remove lymph glands in patients who have no spread. This same technique is used routinely, and successfully, to predict the spread of cancer in people with melanoma.

According to Dr. Khafif, "The concept of a sentinel lymph node is so logical, it is surprising that it has not previously been investigated for breast cancer." People with every type of cancer in which lymph nodes are removed, and people with lymphedema, could not agree more.

phedema, even if he or she has no other surgery at all. And a woman who undergoes a mastectomy with no follow-up radiation may develop lymphedema as a result of the damage the surgery itself does to the lymphatic vessels. Experienced clinicians believe that chemotherapy treatments also increase the risk of getting lymphedema, although exactly how this type of treatment affects the lymphatic system is not clear. It is known, however, that chemotherapy destroys both cancerous and healthy cells, lowers the immune response, and causes a variety of unpleasant symptoms. It may destroy some healthy blood and lymphatic vessels as well. Any subsequent hospitalization or emergency-room visit likewise poses an increased risk of lymphedema—even if these occur years later and for unrelated conditions. Anyone who is facing surgery or other treatment that may result in damage to the lymphatic system should ask his or her doctor *before* being hospitalized about the risk of lymphedema so that precautions can be taken (preventive strategies will be discussed in detail later in this chapter). The ultimate burden of avoiding or managing lymphedema remains with the individual for the rest of his or her life.

OTHER TYPES OF CANCER

While lymph nodes are found throughout the body, they are particularly plentiful in the underarm area, the neck, and the groin. Therefore, anyone undergoing surgery or radiation therapy affecting one or more of these areas is vulnerable to lymphatic damage. In addition, cancer itself can compress and therefore damage blood and lymphatic vessels.

Each year, thousands of women undergo lymph-node removal and/or radiation treatment following surgery for gynecological cancers, procedures including hysterectomy (removal of the uterus), removal of the cervix, and oophorectomy (removal of the ovaries). Lymph nodes are often removed in these procedures. Any woman who undergoes one of these operations is at risk of developing lymphedema in one or both legs. The same is true for men who undergo surgery for prostate cancer, depending upon the stage of the disease and the degree to which it has or may have spread. Even if no lymph nodes are removed, surgery can damage lymphatic vessels. In addition, radiation therapy is often prescribed for men with prostate cancer, and this treatment can further damage lymphatic vessels. Men with advanced testicular cancer that has spread into the lower abdominal area face a similar risk. This spread, or metastasis, of cancer may also happen in cases of colorectal, bladder, pancreatic, and liver cancer. Anyone with any of these conditions is vulnerable to lymphedema as well.

In addition, increasing numbers of individuals each year undergo surgery and lymph-node removal as part of treatment for melanoma, a particularly virulent and systemic cancer of the skin. People with lymphatic damage as a result of these types of cancer (or treatment for them) account for up to 10 percent of lymphedema cases.[6]

ADDITIONAL RISK FACTORS

Contrary to what many people believe, it is not only people whose lymph nodes are found to be cancerous who are vulnerable to lymphedema. Many people have nodes removed that are found to be healthy. Yet they too are at risk for lymphedema because their lymphatic systems have sustained an injury—the removal of lymph nodes. In addition, anyone who has had surgery that caused the development of internal scar tissue can contract the condition, since the formation of such tissue can impede the flow of lymph or block the collateral drainage vessels—vessels in adjacent regions of the body that serve as alternative transport routes, much as you might use a side road to get around a traffic jam on a highway.

In some parts of the world, infection with a tiny parasitic worm called filaria is the most common precursor of lymphedema. The filariae are introduced into the body by the bite of an infected mosquito and migrate to the lymphatic system, where they mature and grow. Eventually, they either block the lymphatic channels or they die and decompose, releasing poisons that cause the lymphatic vessels to become swollen and inflamed. The World Health Organization estimates that 100 million people worldwide have filaritic lymphedema.

Other people at increased risk of developing lymphedema include those with malformations of the veins. Athough rare, this may lead to lymphedema because the blood and lymphatic circulatory systems are so closely related that a problem in the blood system—particularly if surgery has been performed on a vein—may affect the lymphatic system. Also at risk are people who have sustained serious injuries to the lymphatic system as a result of severe accidents or trauma and those who contract infections that interrupt the lymphatic system's normal functioning. While the arms and legs are the most common sites for lymphedema, it can develop in any organ or area of the body, including the face, the abdomen, the lungs, the liver, and the genitals.

A person with lymphedema, whether primary or secondary, may have the condition in only one arm or leg. If you have lower limb lymphedema that affects only one leg, the limb that is not affected must be considered an at-risk limb and treated with preventive measures. Because of the increased risk of infection in a lymphedematous limb, any area of the affected limb that is punctured, scratched, bruised, or injured must be considered endangered as well.

INFECTION

Because damage to the lymphatic system compromises the immune system, people with lymphedema are at increased risk for infections. Since the lymphatic system is an important component of the body's immune system—which functions optimally when lymph flow is unimpeded—the white blood cells and other elements mobilized as part of the immune response become unable to work as they should in fighting infection if the lymphatic system is damaged. In addition, the accumulation of stagnant, protein-rich fluid in the affected arm or leg creates an ideal environment for the proliferation of infection-causing bacteria.

One of the more common types of infection that occur in people with lymphedema is cellulitis, a bacterial infection of the soft tissue of the skin. Cellulitis causes the skin to become red-hot and extremely tender. The redness creeps up the limb and often stops abruptly at the point where the infection ends. Cellulitis is particularly difficult to treat because of its potential and tendency to spread. This type of infection can cause ordinary fluid edema in addition to lymphedema, and edema in turn makes cellulitis even more difficult to treat.

Other types of infection that may occur with lymphedema include lymphangitis (a bacterial infection of the lymphatic channels that most often arises from an area of cellulitis) and lymphadenitis (inflammation of a lymph node that can occur if the node receives lymph from an adjacent infected area). The symptoms of these conditions include swelling, tenderness, pain, and fever.

As we have seen, there are a number of identified risk factors for lymphedema. But remember, risk and onset are two different things. When it comes to onset, there are no hard and fast rules that can predict who will or will not get lymphedema. One person, either during or after an insult to the lymphatic system, may suddenly find his or her arm or leg ballooning. Another may experience slight swelling that is noticeable only because of the tightening of a ring on the finger or difficulty buttoning a sleeve at the wrist. Many people, at least in the early stages of lymphedema, encounter an up-and-down effect.

Because lymphedema is so often neglected and so rarely understood, it is too often attributed to the sufferer—a case of blaming the victim. For instance, it is not uncommon for a person with lymphedema who is overweight to be told that he or she has somehow caused this malady by being heavy. But while obesity can exacerbate the symptoms of lymphedema by placing a strain on the lymphatic vessels, it does not *cause* lymphedema. Similarly, a person who has been stuck by a thorn while gardening or has exercised too strenuously (often without being warned that these activities may be dangerous) may be blamed for the condition.

Always remember that lymphedema is *not* the fault of its sufferers. If anything, it is the "fault" of a damaged lymphatic system and, often, of treatment that is both too little and too late. Any suspicion that lymphedema may be developing should be taken seriously and dealt with aggressively, and anyone who falls into a high-risk category for developing lymphedema should begin immediately to take measures to prevent it.

PREVENTING LYMPHEDEMA

In persons who are at increased risk for developing lymphedema, certain factors, including medical procedures and elements of lifestyle, can increase the risk even further. For example, any penetration of the skin (whether from an injection, a blood-test needle, or a thorn on a rosebush) or constriction or strain on the affected area (whether from a blood-pressure reading, too-tight clothing, or lifting heavy objects) should be avoided. In this section, we will discuss measures the at-risk person can take to reduce his or her risk of developing lymphedema.

If You Require Surgery

By far, the most common causes of lymphedema are removal of lymph nodes and other damage to the lymphatic system as a result of surgery and/or radiation therapy. While there are no surefire strategies to ensure that you will not get lymphedema, you may be able to minimize your risk by learning as much as possible about the condition *before* surgery.

If you are going to the hospital for the first time—having had no prior admissions for surgery—it is a good idea to raise the issue of lymphedema with the hospital admissions clerk. This is the person who formally admits you to the hospital, has you sign permission waivers for various procedures, checks your identification, and makes sure your insurance forms are in order. It is important to have the clerk make an easy-to-see notation on your admitting papers stating that you are having surgery in which lymph nodes may be removed. This request is far from routine, so be prepared for raised eyebrows and, possibly, a less than cooperative response. Don't let that deter you. We believe that only through the individual efforts of patients will hospitals and hospital personnel get the message about the threat that lymphedema poses to people who have lymph nodes removed.

If you have had, or are going to have, surgery that involves the removal of lymph nodes, it is a good idea to carry with you a written warning, such as the following:

I AM AT RISK FOR LYMPHEDEMA BECAUSE I HAVE HAD (OR MAY HAVE) MY LYMPH NODES REMOVED. THEREFORE, NO BLOOD SAMPLES ARE TO BE DRAWN, NO BLOOD-PRESSURE READINGS TAKEN, AND NO NEEDLES USED ON MY AFFECTED ARM, HAND, OR LEG.

Sign your name at the bottom of the warning, and keep several copies with you at all times, clipped to your health-insurance card. Whenever you enter a hospital or doctor's office, discuss your warning with the admitting clerk, nurse, and doctor. If there is no time for discussion, simply request that it be placed in your medical record or chart. Do not leave this to chance; specifically request that a note be added to your record or chart—underlined in red—to alert all members of your health-care team to your situation. In addition, give a copy of your warning to someone who is close to you, preferably the person who accompanies you to the hospital. Enlist that person's help in reinforcing your warnings, or in making a bold sign restating the warnings to be taped to the head of your bed.

Immediately before surgery, a doctor or nurse will insert an intravenous (IV) line in your arm. This provides the route through which fluids and/or medications will be administered. Make sure to tell the person who performs this procedure *not* to start an IV in the arm on the side of your body that the surgery will be, since any puncturing of the skin creates potential for bacteria to enter and infection to result. If both arms are affected, this procedure can be done in a leg. Also, make sure that the person who starts your IV line makes a prominent note on your chart as a reminder to other hospital personnel who may care for you.

Before surgery, your anesthesiologist will probably meet with you. This is the time to tell him or her of your concern about contracting lymphedema; it is the anesthesiologist who will monitor your IV during surgery and who may start a new IV line if the existing one must be replaced.

You should not allow any blood samples to be taken from an affected arm or hand, nor should injections be given in that arm or hand. If the lymphedema affects a leg or legs, no injections should be given into any part of either leg or into the buttocks. This caveat applies to vaccinations as well as to other injections.

Another procedure that you can count on being performed with some frequency, both before and after surgery, is blood-pressure testing. Hospital personnel routinely take blood-pressure readings from a person's "free" arm—that is, the one with no IV in it. However, if you have had surgery in which underarm lymph nodes have been removed and/or the lymphatic vessels disturbed, you should insist that blood-pressure readings *not* be taken from the affected arm. This is because the pressure the cuff exerts pushes the fluid in your arm upward and downward—like the air in a balloon being squeezed in the middle—and it puts you at greater risk of developing lymphedema. Harmless as this painless, one-minute-or-less procedure has always been in the past, it now poses a threat.

One reason why it is so important to have a warning note in your medical chart is that, most often, blood-pressure readings and blood samples are taken immediately after surgery, when you may be too groggy from anesthesia to object. Sometimes these procedures are performed in the middle of the night, when you are either sleeping or too drowsy to say anything. Without the written warning, the person caring for you may have no way of knowing that an arm or leg is off-limits. In addition, while you are in the hospital, you may find that the person attending to your care one day is not the same person who cares for you the next day. Hospitals have three shifts—day, evening, and night—and personnel rotations are common. Even a nurse or doctor who has been alerted may forget your warnings, so continued vigilance is paramount.

If, for some reason, blood pressure must be taken on an affected arm—for instance, if there are multiple IVs in the other arm or if you have undergone a double mastectomy—ask the person taking the reading to use the cuff, not one of the newer digital machines. The new devices remain on the arm for a longer period of time, placing pressure on your arm's already strained vessels and possibly weakening or destroying them—or even bringing about lymphedema.

It is important to be alert to the changes in hospital personnel that have taken place in this country over the past few years. As health care has become increasingly driven by corporate economic decisions, many hospitals have downsized their registered-nurse staffs and replaced RNs with unlicensed, minimally trained aides and technicians. Because few hospital personnel now wear name pins that identify their professional status, patients often do not know who is attending to their needs. Do not hesitate to ask any person who is attending to you if he or she is a medical doctor or registered nurse. Only MDs and RNs are clinically trained to assess your condition, including the most subtle signs that may indicate the onset of lymphedema. It is your right to request that only an RN or MD take your blood pressure or give you an injection.

The need for vigilance on the part of the hospitalized patient that all of these precautions create cannot be overstated. After surgery, patients have to deal with physical discomfort, emotional ups and downs, mental stress, and the unfamiliar disturbance of hospital routine. Having to remember to check your caregiver's credentials

The Pink Wristband

The pink wristband is a simple device used to signify that an arm (or leg) is either affected by or at risk of developing lymphedema. Already in use in a number of hospitals across the United States, the pink wristband is identical to the red wristband commonly used to alert medical personnel to a patient's potentially life-threatening allergies. It is a flat, adjustable plastic band that looks like all other hospital identification bracelets. Ideally, it should be about eight to ten inches long and no more than three-quarters inch wide (leg or ankle bands should of course be wider). It should be a bright, hot pink—a color that is noticeable on all skin tones, stands out, and is easily recognizable. The band should also be latex-free, since many people are allergic to latex. And it should be clearly imprinted with the following warning: NO BLOOD PRESSURE, IV, OR INJECTION ON THIS ARM (OR LEG). Some hospitals have purchased pink wristbands with preprinted warnings; others write the warnings themselves.

If you have lymphedema, you should wear the band or carry it with you at all times. This is important because even if your limb appears relatively normal, it may contain an accumulation of stagnant, protein-rich fluid that predisposes you to infection, a constant risk especially in hospitals. If you do not have lymphedema but have had surgery that involved lymph-node removal, wear the pink wristband as long as you are in the hospital and also for all subsequent hospital admissions and doctor visits.

If you know you are going to be hospitalized, call or visit the chief executive or nursing administrator of the hospital ahead of time and ask whether they routinely issue pink wristbands for patients who have or are at risk for lymphedema. If they do not, ask that they create a pink wristband for you. If they are unfamiliar with the concept, explain that you need a band that is identical to the standard red allergy band, except that it should be pink in color.

If your hospital does not or cannot supply you with a pink wristband, you can buy one on your own (see the Resources section at the end of the book for more information). Or you can fashion one for yourself by cutting a strip of bright pink fabric or paper, writing the warnings on it, covering it with a soft plastic coating, stitching the ends closed, then attaching small pieces of velcro on the ends to allow you to close it. Or you can bring the strip of fabric or paper with you to the hospital and ask the person who puts on your hospital bracelet to put the pink wristband on as well.

Upon admission to the hospital, put on the pink wristband and do not remove it until you leave. If you have had bilateral breast surgery, wear two pink wristbands, one on each wrist. Explain to all of your caretakers what the pink wristband means: "Do not take blood pressure, start IVs, or give injections in this arm or hand!" If you are at risk for lower limb lymphedema, the pink wristband will serve as a constant reminder to both you and the hospital staff that you are at risk, and that the appropriate precautions—such as not giving injections into the buttocks—must be taken. If it is necessary to remove the band for any reason, it should be replaced immediately, before you are moved to another site—a laboratory for tests, a new unit, a lounge, or your room.

After surgery, if you are undergoing chemotherapy by injection or by an intravenous route, wear the pink wristband on the affected limb to make sure the medication is not administered into that limb. Wear the pink wristband every day or carry it with you at all times. Also, buy a MedicAlert bracelet or necklace that includes the fact that you have lymphedema and the instructions: "No IVs, blood pressure, or injections in affected limb." (See the Resources section at the end of this book for further information.)

Will a pink wristband cure lymphedema? No. Will it prevent it? Possibly. There are no guarantees, but wearing the band will help to prevent mistakes from being made in the one place you should feel most safe—the hospital. It can also serve as an educational tool, inspiring hospitals to train their staff to educate at-risk patients about the precautions they must take for the rest of their lives.

or to warn bedside personnel to avoid taking blood pressure, drawing blood samples, or giving injections in your affected limb may seem like one burden too many. But it's worth it!

Usually, requests of this kind are accommodated, and whoever is attending you will say, "Oh, your other arm—well, whichever arm you prefer." But some personnel may try to dismiss your concerns, saying that "research hasn't proven" a relationship between lymphedema and blood-pressure readings, blood samples, or injections. Unfortunately, medical history is full of examples of dangers being proven only after large numbers of people were harmed. DES, a drug once given to pregnant women to prevent miscarriage; the Dalkon Shield and Copper 7 intrauterine devices (IUDs); and silicone breast implants all were utilized in great quantities before they were either taken off the market or their use modified because of safety concerns. So the "research hasn't proven" argument is one you cannot afford to lose. Insist, make a fuss if you have to, and if that doesn't work, refuse any procedure until your doctor writes an order that respects your wishes. It is your legal right to do this. Always keep in mind that you are trying to avoid a condition that has no cure, few treatments, and, once acquired, lasts a lifetime.

What if you absolutely need surgery on an at-risk limb—or, worse, a limb already affected by lymphedema? Obviously, this presents a threat to the person who fears exacerbating lymphedema's symptoms and making the condition worse. If you need any kind of surgery on an affected limb—or on any other part of your body, for that matter—it is a good idea to have your surgeon consult with your lymphedema therapist (lymphedema therapy will be discussed in Chapter 3). In this way, your doctor can learn what your lymphedema therapy has involved, what the implications of disturbing your already compromised lymphatic system are, and how to avoid doing so—or at least how to minimize the risk of further damage.

No surgeon should take exception to this kind of help. As with all specialists, surgeons focus on their particular area of expertise, rather than on its aftermath or possible "side effects." It goes without saying that many people who now have lymphedema might have avoided it had their surgeons appreciated the drastic long-term effects of lymphatic damage and/or consulted beforehand with experts in lymphedema. So if you need surgery, don't hesitate to ask your doctor and lymphedema therapist to speak with each other. It may save you years of grief.

If You Require Chemotherapy, Radiation Therapy, or Hormonal Therapy

For people with cancer, treatment does not end after surgery has been performed—as anyone who has been through follow-up radiation therapy, chemotherapy, or hormonal therapy knows. These treatments, known as adjuvant therapies, are commonly recommended after cancer surgery to destroy any remaining cancer cells that may have traveled to other parts of the body. In some cases, they are given before surgery as well to shrink tumors or prevent cancer from spreading.

Radiation therapy is among the most common pre- and post-surgery treatments in this country. Although most people wince when they hear the word *radiation*, there are several positive things to say about radiation treatments. They usually have tolerable and manageable side effects, they are usually over in six to eight weeks, and, most important, they bombard and destroy any remaining cancer cells that may exist. However, they may also cause fatigue, swelling, soreness, and redness or discoloration, and, as we have seen, they increase the risk of lymphedema.

If you must undergo radiation therapy, you should examine the area being treated daily and apply a soothing and protective ointment recommended by your doctor to any reddened areas of skin. You should also scrupulously avoid exposure to sunlight and avoid chlorinated pools, hot tubs, and hot showers. Be alert for any danger signals—a ring or shoe that becomes too tight, a feeling of heaviness in the arm or leg, or changes in the appearance of the skin, for example—and bring these signs to your doctor's attention immediately.

Chemotherapy—which literally means "therapy with chemicals," is a systemic drug therapy that may be recommended following cancer surgery. It involves the administration of one or more very toxic drugs to kill cancerous cells and is done over a period of anywhere from six months to several years. Chemotherapy agents may be taken by mouth or administered by injection or intravenously. Some types of chemotherapy are given in the doctor's office, others in the hospital during a stay of one or several nights. If you are receiving chemotherapy either by injection or by intravenous transfusion, remember to wear a pink wristband on your affected arm as a reminder that medical personnel are not to administer the drugs in that limb.

The repeated injections or IV infusions of chemotherapy may damage the veins, further compromising the circulatory system. If an IV in an unaffected arm no longer functions properly, those administering the treatment may decide to start an IV in the affected arm. To avoid this, ask them to do it in a leg or consider asking for a mediport, a surgically implanted device that has a plug designed to accept an intravenous line, for as long as your chemotherapy treatments continue. A mediport may be implanted in the chest or an unaffected arm. The surgery to implant it can be done on an outpatient basis in many cases, but it does require general anesthesia, and it may take two to three weeks for the area to heal before the mediport can be used, so advance planning may be necessary.

Lowered resistance to infection, a result of bone-marrow suppression, is another problem that occurs with cancer chemotherapy, and it can be especially dangerous to the person at risk for lymphedema. Skin rashes, dryness, and cracking (particularly in or near the underarm or groin area, or on the affected arm or leg) are not uncommon side effects of chemotherapy, and can cause inflammation and the threat of infection, which the body may be unable to fight off. Because of the threat of infection during chemotherapy, it is important not only to employ the ordinary preventive strategies we have suggested in this chapter, but also to wear a mask in crowded public places, avoid socializing with people who have colds, stay away from children who have recently received immunizations, and avoid eating fresh fruits and vegetables, as they may be full of bacteria (eat your vegetables steamed or canned instead). It is also a good idea to seek the advice of a licensed nutritionist, preferably one who works with an oncologist. Nutritionists can be extremely helpful in recommending nutrients (in foods or in supplement form) that can help you maintain your nutritional status, boost your immune system, and possibly avoid the onset of lymphedema.

Hormonal therapy also raises a number of issues related to lymphedema. Because the growth of some breast cancers appears to be associated with the presence of the sex hormone estrogen, your doctor may prescribe a hormone-suppressing agent after surgery. Probably the best known of these agents is tamoxifen (Nolvadex), a nonsteroidal anti-estrogen originally synthesized in 1966. Some studies have found this drug to be effective in preventing the recurrence of breast cancer, and it may also decrease both blood cholesterol and the risk of osteoporosis. However, it does have some effects that should be of concern to women who have, or who are at risk of developing, lymphedema.[7]

First, tamoxifen can cause water retention and weight gain in some people. This type of water retention is the high-sodium type, or ordinary edema, not the high-protein swelling of lymphedema. However, any fluid retention places a strain on the circulatory system, so if you must take this medication, you should adhere strictly to a low-salt, low-protein diet, avoid becoming overheated, and take other measures for alleviating ordinary water retention (more about this in Chapter 7).

Rarely, inflammation of the blood vessels and the formation of blood clots in the veins have been linked to tamoxifen therapy. If you take tamoxifen and have or are at risk for lymphedema, you should be alert to symptoms of thromboembolitic (blood-clot-related) disease. These include swelling of an arm or leg; pain or warmth in an arm or leg; shortness of breath that comes on abruptly; chest pain; or coughing and spitting up blood. If any of these symptoms develops, seek medical help at once.

Other Cautionary Measures

Once you are at risk for lymphedema, you must make changes—forever—in the way you do certain very ordinary things. You should, in fact, observe the same precautions as a person who already has the condition, including not straining or compressing the affected limb and taking meticulous care of your skin. Lymphedema calls for numerous changes in your everyday life—really, a whole new lifestyle. This will be discussed in detail in Chapter 6.

Lymphedema is the proverbial horse behind the cart, most often occurring *after* extensive and often complicated surgery or other treatments. Typically, a person who complains of heaviness or swelling in a limb after such treatment is told that this is an inevitable byproduct of surgery and that the best solution is to learn to live with it. We have heard about (and from) many people who have undergone cancer surgery who report that their doctors minimized the symptoms of lymphedema by telling them that they should feel lucky to be alive. It is our opinion that doctors should be held accountable for neglecting to inform their patients of all the risks involved in their treatment, including the risk of lymphedema, as well as for failing to implement or suggest effective treatments in a timely fashion. It is your right to know!

Prevention is immeasurably better than treatment for this incurable condition. If you think a diagnostic, surgical, or radiation treatment, or a traumatic accident, has put you at risk for lymphedema, you should discuss this concern with your doctor. And feel free to share with your doctor what you have learned about the prevention and treatment of lymphedema. No one, not even doctors, knows everything, and your information may be greatly appreciated and utilized to provide better treatment for you and other patients. Once you start to think of yourself as a potential candidate for lymphedema and start to address its risks, you will be well on your way to preventing the condition—or, if despite your best efforts, it does develop, to managing it effectively.

Part II

Treatment

Introduction

People experiencing the first symptoms of lymphedema are likely to be bewildered, and their questions come tumbling out: "What do I have? How did I get it? Is there any treatment that can help me? Now what should I do?" They want the doctor to do something—anything—to make the swelling go away.

Once lymphedema is diagnosed, either by your doctor or by you, effective, long-lasting treatment becomes the goal. But since the condition has not received its fair share of attention—in the media, through word of mouth, or even in the medical and scientific-research communities—learning about the treatments that exist is not always easy. For example, despite its widespread incidence, lymphedema is not included in the otherwise comprehensive medical sections of the encyclopedias featured on various Internet sites. If you try to look up *lymphedema* in the dictionary—even an unabridged dictionary—chances are you won't find it. Before this book was published, there were no books devoted exclusively to the condition. There has been a serious lack of research studies on the subject, particularly in this country. Even the U.S. Centers for Disease Control and Prevention in Atlanta has no data on the prevalence or incidence of lymphedema.[1]

Just as there are no standard criteria for diagnosis, there are none for treatment. Many people seeking help find that their doctors are not informed about lymphedema or the lifelong problems it poses if neglected. They may simply be told to elevate the limb, only to find this recommendation works for just a short time—if at all. Some people may be told to use a pump, others to find a massage therapist, yet others to wrap the swollen limb with stretch bandages.

Today, a variety of therapies are available, some more effective than others. In this section we will discuss the conventional and alternative treatments that are most commonly employed, including a regimen known as complete decongestive physiotherapy (CDP), which appears to offer the best and most long-lasting relief for lymphedema at this time. We will also look at the different types of practitioners and facilities you may choose to provide treatment, and discuss what to look for when choosing someone to treat your lymphedema.

3
Conventional Treatment

After being diagnosed with lymphedema, you will no doubt be eager for relief and willing to enter treatment, even if that treatment requires time and expense. You may already have tried elevating your limb without getting any relief, and your symptoms may be getting worse. When you return to your doctor for additional advice, you may be told, "Elevation is just about the only treatment I can suggest. Try doing it more often."

Since an accumulation of fluid is the basic problem in lymphedema, many people's first question is, Why not just drain the fluid, as doctors do for water on the knee? Unfortunately, this is not an option because lymphatic fluid accumulates within the tissues and therefore is not in a single location from which it might be drained.

There is no cure for lymphedema, and no sure way to prevent it—at least not at this time. In spite of all the preventive measures people may take, many thousands still develop this condition each year. Nevertheless, treatments do exist that have proven helpful to lymphedema sufferers around the world. By finding the treatment you need, you will start on the path to effective management of your condition. Remember, lymphedema is a lifelong condition, so management, not cure, is the ultimate goal.

The treatments used for lymphedema today are significantly more effective than some of the esoteric measures used in the past.[1] In some European countries, for instance, it used to be common to "wring out" lymphatic fluid from the affected limb with a rubber tube, using more pressure than is used in typical blood-pressure readings. This procedure was so painful that it was often performed under general anesthesia, and it was so risky that both tissues and remaining lymphatic vessels were often damaged. In mesotherapy, which was first described in medical literature in 1958 and is still used in some European countries, a drug mixture is injected into the tissues by means of a gunlike device that contains numerous small needles. This technique is used to treat the pain of arthritis, migraine headaches, cellulitis, and vascular diseases. The standard drugs used include very small quantities of the anesthetic procaine or lidocaine, vitamin B_1 or B_{12}, and sometimes an antibiotic or a vaso-dilator (a drug that relaxes and dilates the blood vessels). In lymphedema therapy, an enzyme is added to the mixture to break down protein. However, this treatment is of doubtful benefit and it can cause tissue damage. Moreover, the safety of the drugs that are used is open to question.

If your doctor is knowledgeable about lymphedema treatment, he or she may have already suggested one—or all—of the treatments that are discussed in this chapter. Or you may be reading about such treatment here for the very first time. All of the treatments discussed here have a degree of effectiveness. But since each one serves a different need, you have the best chance of being helped if your treatment includes a combination of therapies.

PUMPS

One treatment for lymphedema involves the use of a pump, a table-top device that can be placed on an end table or night table. Sequential pumps, developed in the mid-1990s, force compressed air into succeeding segments of a sleeve that fits over the entire length of the affected limb. Pumps used as recently as five years ago squeezed the entire limb at one time. While these are still on the market, they are less effective than today's gradient pumps and, in some cases, are even damaging, so they should not be used.

There are two types of sequential pumps available. The standard sequential compression system is a multichamber pump that applies the same pressure to each section of the garment in turn. The peristaltic gradient compression system more closely mimics the natural pressure changes in the limb that normally power the movement of lymph through the lymphatic vessels. This device consists of air-compression pumps, a pneumatic garment divided into sections, and air hoses that connect the pump to individual compartments of the garment. Once the limb is placed in the garment and the machine turned on, the sequential gradient pump provides continuous pneumatic compression to gently massage or "milk" the lymphatic vessels of the arm or leg, forcing large amounts of fluid from the limb into unaffected areas of the body, from which it can drain normally.

The garment provides peristaltic action up the limb; the first chamber inflates and holds, followed by the second chamber. When the third chamber inflates, the first one deflates, and so on. This sequential compression provides continuous pressure where needed while relieving unnecessary pressure on tissues behind the wave of compression. For lymphedema of the leg, it works best if the person using it is lying down; for lymphedema of the arm, it works best if the arm is elevated. But even though compression can remove fluid, it cannot remove protein (remember that lymphedema is characterized by the accumulation of protein and fat molecules as well as fluid). Protein left behind in the tissues may become fibrotic, forming minute, scarlike obstacles that impede the lymphatic fluid's flow. In addition, if a pump is used on a continual basis, fluid and protein may leak out of the lymphatic system and back into the tissues of the trunk of the body, causing a buildup of excess fluid and fibrotic deposits in the shoulder area (in arm lymphedema) or in the unaffected leg or groin area (in leg lymphedema). In effect, the fluid may be pushed out of the limb but end up accumulating at whatever location the pumping is terminated. If this happens, it can further compromise an already limited lymphatic system.

There are other downsides to the pump as well. An Australian study on the use of the pump in lymphedema therapy involved 1,036 lymphedema patients, 402 of whom had used the pump in treatment and assessed its effects themselves. Of these individuals, 199 noted some improvement. However, the incidence of complications increased from 13 to 32 percent in people with lymphedema of the arm, and from 30 to 55 percent in people with lymphedema of the leg. These complications were not minor. They included the development of lymphedema in previously normal genitalia, trunks, or opposite limbs; the formation of scar tissue; and bruising and aching of the treated limb. Researchers concluded that sequential pumps yielded more improvements than single-chambered pumps did, but also were associated with more complications.[2]

In another study, patients with leg lymphedema were studied by trained observers in a U.S. treatment center. In one group, two of fifty-five patients experienced genital lymphedema before pump therapy, but use of the pump actually *caused* this devastating condition in twenty-three others. The researchers pointed out that the incidence of genital lymphedema among this group of patients was not affected by age or sex; the duration or severity of the lymphedema; the cause of the condition; or whether one or both legs were affected.[3]

Pumps cost many thousands of dollars. They can be bought or rented from manufacturers or medical-supply stores, and lymphedema patients often use pumps at home. However, there is some debate among lymphedema specialists about whether or not pumps should be used in the home, since there is always the risk of a layperson misusing a pump and further injuring his or her lymphatic system. Most experts in lymphedema therapy feel that pumps should never be used at home.[4] In addition, Medicare guidelines now require anyone who uses a pump to provide extensive documentation, including a treatment plan and ongoing monitoring, in order to qualify for Medicare coverage. This is difficult to do outside a treatment facility.

Unfortunately, it is not uncommon for a doctor to recommend a pump, or even to hand one over to a patient, with little or no instruction as to how to use it, leaving the patient to figure it out—as if he or she were purchasing a VCR. The mistakes that you can make in setting a VCR, however, have little consequence. Misuse of the pump can have disastrous consequences. Many people who have been handed a pump without instructions return home and crank up the pump pressure so high that damage to the remaining lymphatic vessels ensues.

Therefore, if you decide to try using a pump on your own, it is absolutely essential that you be instructed by a doctor, lymphedema therapist, or trained technician as to the proper use of the device and also about problems that may arise. Do not just pick up a pump at a medical-supply store or your doctor's office, take it home, and try to figure it out on your own. And never lend the pump to a friend. Each person has a different tolerance for the pump's pressure, and some people have coexisting conditions, such as cardiac problems, high blood pressure, and other ailments, that make the use of a pump inadvisable or that may have to be closely monitored by a medical doctor.

Once you know how to use the pump correctly, you must determine the amount of pressure you can tolerate. Protocols for using pumps vary, and there does not appear to be a consensus either in medical literature or among the medical community as to which pumps are most effective, at what pressure, and for what duration. However, a general rule of thumb is that you should not experience any pain or uncomfortable pressure. Again, you should count on a professional to instruct you. Most important, the gradient pump must be used immediately after the first sign of swelling—discomfort or a lack of normal mobility in the limb—when the arm or leg is least likely to have fibrotic protein deposits, which further impair lymph flow. However, you should be aware that there are situations in which a pump should never be used:

• If you have primary lymphedema. The pump is not recommended at all in such cases because it can cause lymphedema of the genital area, leakage of fluid from the skin, and swelling in the normal limb.

• If you have blood-vessel disease or severe arteriosclerosis, massive edema from congestive heart failure, deformity of the limb, or metastatic cancer in the involved limb.

• If you have dermatitis, gangrene, recent skin grafts, deep venous thrombosis (blood clots in the veins), or—especially—cellulitis.

If for any reason the pump gives you a problem, bring it to your doctor or lymphedema therapist immediately and explain exactly what the problem is. He or she may be able to solve the problem, or it may be advisable for you to discontinue use of the device.

Clearly, pump therapy is not a cure-all. There is such a widespread lack of instruction from medical professionals as to how to use pumps properly that many lymphedema patients either abandon pump therapy because it yields little progress or, even when used in good faith, further damages the lymphatic system. Ironically, however, it is often the only treatment that insurance companies cover. (A discussion of insurance coverage for lymphedema treatment will be found in Chapter 10). For the long-term management of lymphedema, the pump alone is not as effective as is a combination of therapies that also includes manual lymph drainage, massage, and wrapping (information about these therapies will be found later in this chapter). However, this complex treatment is expensive and time-consuming and, in many locations, simply unavailable. If there is no lymphedema treatment center or therapist in your area, the pump can be a viable alternative—used only after proper training, of course. Family members, friends, or you yourself can be trained to use the pump and administer massage.

LYMPHEDEMA THERAPY

To judge by the numbers of people who suffer for years before they succeed in finding help, or who give up looking because their efforts are unsuccessful, you would think that lymphedema is a rare or recent phenomenon. Nothing could be further from the truth. People have always suffered from the effects of damaged lymphatic systems and tried to find relief. Although lymphedema therapy has been a staple of European medical practice for well over a century, it has found its way to the United States only in the last several years.

Over 100 years ago, a German doctor, A. von Winiwarter, first used a type of physical therapy or massage known as manual lymph drainage (MLD) to treat lymphedema. This method was improved by a Danish physician, Emil Vodder, and his wife, Estrid, in the 1930s, and the Vodders' method was in turn refined by their protégés, particularly an Austrian couple, Hildegard and Guenther Wittlinger, and their son, Dieter. The practice of manual lymph drainage became widespread, and it is now used by certified practitioners around the world. These professionals are considered among the most adept and knowledgeable in the field of lymphedema treatment. In the 1980s, two German doctors, Michael and Ethel Foeldi, improved the drainage technique further, and it was subsequently refined by two pioneering Australian practitioners, the late John R. Casley-Smith, DSc, MD, and Judith R. Casley-Smith, MA, PhD, internationally recognized experts in lymphedema and founders of the Australian Lymphoedema Association.

It can be hard for patients to make sense of the alphabet soup of terms used to describe lymphedema therapies. In the 1930s, when Dr. Vodder developed his lymphedema treatment technique, it was called complex decongestive physiotherapy (CDP), and it included skin cleansing and MLD. Many lymphedema therapists and teachers have taken the lead of the Casley-Smiths, who called their treatment complex physical therapy (CPT). CPT includes not only scrupulous skin cleansing and MLD but also bandaging, the wearing of a compression garment, and exercise.

The terms CDP, CPT, and MLD are often, but erroneously, used interchangeably to describe lymphedema treatment. Actually, MLD is only *one* of the treatments that help lymphedema patients attain their ultimate goal. MLD cannot bring about long-lasting relief unless it is combined with the other facets of lymphedema treatment, namely skin cleansing, bandaging, exercise, and the wearing of a compression garment.

Today, with increasing numbers of physicians and researchers recognizing the importance and widespread nature of lymphedema, treatment is appropriately called CDP/MLD, and practitioners who have studied and become certified in these techniques often place these letters after their names. Most people who study CDP and MLD in the United States must spend at least two weeks learning the techniques, although there are no U.S. standards mandating hours of study or other requirements for certification (in Europe, in contrast, there is a minimum requirement of 135 to 150 hours of study). Whatever the treatment is called, however, it involves the full participation of patient, therapist, and doctor, and the goal is the same: to open up collateral, or secondary, lymphatic vessels so that the limbs with edema can drain into normally functioning tributaries. This brings about maximum lymphatic drainage and long-lasting relief of symptoms.

Manual Lymph Drainage

Manual lymph drainage (MLD) is the common name given to a massage technique used to treat lymphedema. Today, it is often used as part of complete decongestive physiotherapy (CDP).

Phase one of CDP treatment, used to treat acute flare-ups, must be done by a professional. Treatment is usually given once or twice a day over a period of two to four weeks. It involves gentle massage followed by wrapping with low-stretch bandages, under which foam padding or gauze is applied, and specific exercises recommended by the lymphedema therapist. In phase two, the maintenance stage, you can apply the massage techniques at home, put on the compression garment independently, and continue the exercises. In cases of primary lymphedema affecting infants who are too young for comprehensive therapy (with wrapping and compression garments), massage alone can be extremely effective and can often be performed by the parents.

Gentle is a key concept in MLD. This type of light-touch massage, when applied to the skin surface, prevents damage to the skin and tissues and aids the flow of lymph through the superficial lymphatic vessels beneath the skin into areas of the circulatory system that drain normally. (In people with lymphedema, the superficial vessels are likely to be working normally; the problem usually lies in the deeper vessels.) Occasionally, the massage is moderately vigorous, such as when the therapist's goal is to force fluid through tissue in which scar tissue has formed. But more forceful massage runs the risk of damaging lymphatic vessels, overloading adjacent lymphatic vessels, and encouraging the development of even more high-protein scar tissue.

The rhythmic massage of MLD is conducted segmentally—the therapist works on one section of the limb at a time, then goes to an adjacent section, moving from the affected area to the unaffected area and always in the direction of lymph flow—that is, toward the body. If the limb with lymphedema is too sensitive or sore to withstand massage in the early stages of treatment, the unaffected side is massaged first. Because increasing circulation in one part of the body stimulates the circulation in all the other parts, this helps to improve the flow of lymph and open up superficial lymphatic vessels on the affected side. This is often necessary for people who have lipedema, a condition characterized by swelling and abnormal deposition of adipose (fatty) tissue in the legs. This condition occurs mostly in women. A person with lipedema may have a slim upper body, but legs that are many times their normal size, vulnerable to bruising, and extremely sensitive to touch. Because the fat deposits in the legs block the flow of lymphatic fluid, lipedema often leads to the development of lymphedema—which, unfortunately, is rarely diagnosed and therefore rarely treated. If lymphedema is diagnosed, people with lipedema can obtain great relief of pain, a reduction of swelling in their limbs, and a reduction in fatty deposits with MLD.

Complete Decongestive Physiotherapy

Complete decongestive physiotherapy is a product of the work of the late John R. Casley-Smith, MD, and his wife Judith R. Casley-Smith, PhD (see page 48). The Casley-Smiths conducted extensive research on lymphedema and its treatment, and have trained hundreds of CDP practitioners. In an American study done in 1994, the Casley-Smiths reported significant reductions in lymphedematous limbs with the CDP technique, and cited additional successes with the method in Australia, Switzerland, and Germany.[5] In the American study, they followed thirty-eight lymphedema patients, most of them female, who ranged in age from two to eighty-two. Thirteen had primary lymphedema and twenty-five had secondary lymphedema, among them sixteen who had lymphedema as a result of breast-cancer surgery. The multilevel treatment they received took four hours a day and lasted thirty days, and included the following:

• First, the therapist cleansed and lubricated the subject's skin. Any dead tissue was removed, and antibiotic ointments were applied.

• Second, the therapist applied manual pressure to bring fluid from the swollen areas into the "watershed" area of the body—the abdominal area, where fluid is plentiful. This redirected the flow of lymphatic fluid toward healthy lymphatic vessels and opened up the healthy vessels.

• Third, the therapist placed gauze bags filled with chips of latex over the fibrotic (scarred) areas, then wrapped layers of stocking bandages on the affected limbs. This increased tissue pressure, broke down the scar tissue and prevented the stagnating lymphatic fluid from returning to the limbs. The subjects wore the wrapping throughout the course of therapy.

• Finally, the therapist developed an individualized program of exercises that improved muscular contractions and joint mobility, strengthened the affected limbs, and helped to reduce the atrophy of muscles.

In this study, subjects with upper limb lymphedema showed an average 73-percent reduction in swelling as a result of the therapy. Among the eighteen patients with lymphedema of one leg, there was an 88-percent reduction in swelling. After twelve months the reduction remained in all but two patients. Some patients later experienced partial relapses because they failed to wear their compression garments, but their lymphedema never returned to pretreatment levels. In another study, published in 1997, Drs. Marvin Boris and Stanley Weindorf, together with physical therapist Bonnie Lasinski, found that patients who received CDP maintained either a partial or complete reduction in swelling after three years and showed 100-percent compliance with the treatment.[6]

Not every practitioner of lymphedema therapy follows exactly the same regimen. For example, some cleanse the skin first but lubricate it after the massage is administered. Often there is no need to remove any dead tissue. In general, however, you can expect a lymphedema therapist to begin by cleansing and lubricating the skin, then performing the gentle massage of manual lymph drainage. After MLD is performed, the therapist wraps the affected limb with bandages that exert greatest compression at the farthest end (the hand or foot), with decreasing pressure as the bandages go toward the trunk. These low-stretch bandages act as a second skin, providing constant counterpressure to the muscular contractions that keep the lymphatic fluid moving along. In essence, wrapping (or bandaging) is similar to mummifying. It helps the muscles in the limb to pump the lymphedematous fluid in much the same way electronic or manual pumps do.

It is helpful to learn how to apply the bandages yourself, particularly for times when you take long airplane trips or exercise, since changes in cabin pressure and/or exertion can cause the limb to swell.

Wrapping is done each day for up to four weeks, and the bandages stay on the affected limb twenty-four hours a day. The process is repeated with each treatment until the arm or leg shows a significant reduction in swelling. Often, hard foam-rubber padding or gauze chips are placed under the wrapping to increase pressure on particular spots. This helps to soften or shape the area and break down any scar tissue that has developed.

Each day, when the bandages are removed, you take a shower, after which the therapist checks your limb for any breaks in the skin or signs of infection, and the degree of swelling is assessed. If there is any opening in the skin—something that might lead to an infection such as cellulitis—or any red marks are apparent, your therapist will apply a topical antibiotic such as mupirocin (Bactroban) before the limb is rebandaged. He or she may also apply a lotion or lotions to soften the skin.

Some therapists have been experimenting with the use of emu oil as a skin lubricant for people with lymphedema. This oil is nontoxic, and has antibacterial, antimicrobial, and antiinflammatory properties, in addition to being an excellent moisturizer and emollient. Many lymphedema therapists have found that the damaging effects on the skin of radiation therapy are greatly helped by the application of emu oil.

Sometimes, with upper limb lymphedema, the arm is wrapped with a low-stretch dressing covered with a plastic covering that is secured by tape at the wrist, elbow, and upper arm. This allows the person to take a shower at home and do light household chores without getting the dressing wet. One inventive businessman we know saw his wife wearing this plastic-covered protection and bought her a pair of deer-dressing gloves that went up to the shoulder. Wearing these gloves, his wife was able to shower and do dishes and other light chores with comfort and complete protection against water. Deer-dressing gloves can be bought at many sporting-goods stores.

CDP is done for four to eight weeks or until a reduction in

swelling is achieved. There are several advantages to complete decongestive physiotherapy:

• It is noninvasive.

• It establishes collateral lymphatic-vessel pathways that remain open.

• It gradually and gently reroutes the stagnant lymphatic fluid from the swollen limb into the circulatory system.

• It stimulates a damaged or weakened lymphatic system.

• It dilates the lymphatic vessels so they can handle increasing amounts of fluid.

• It softens areas of scarring.

• It reduces medical expenses. (While CDP is expensive, it is not nearly as expensive as going for *years* to numerous doctors—dermatologists, internists, psychiatrists, and others—for treatment of the various physical and psychological symptoms of lymphedema.)

• It brings about better functioning of the affected limb and the lymphatic system.

• It allows you to feel better and more in control of your treatment.

During pregnancy, when blood volume and other body fluids normally expand, a woman should undergo lymphedema therapy only after she has consulted with her obstetrician, a vascular specialist, and an expert in lymphedema therapy.

COMPRESSION GARMENTS

Another treatment your lymphedema therapist is likely to suggest is a compression sleeve or stocking. Actually, this is not so much a treatment as it is a part of daily life for the person with lymphedema, on a par with dentures or eyeglasses or a hearing aid. As we have seen, lymphatic drainage is only part of effective and long-lasting treatment. Wearing a compression garment is paramount for maximum success in reducing swelling and making sure that it stays reduced.

The compression sleeve or stocking is not an elastic bandage. Rather, it is a tightly knit one-piece elasticized cotton garment, similar to the type of stockings that are worn for varicose veins.

Both arm and leg sleeves are open at both ends, except for arm sleeves that include handpieces. They are usually beige-colored, but some manufacturers make sleeves in various fashion colors as well as in black and white. A compression garment must never be worn on an untreated, swollen limb because it will not, by itself, reduce swelling. Treatment with a pump and/or manual lymph drainage should be undertaken before a compression garment is used.

For swelling of the scrotum in men, there are specially made compression garments that can provide relief. If genital swelling occurs in a child or teenager, a jockstrap may be helpful if the compression garment is too binding.

Getting the Proper Fit

Like any garment, the sleeve should be properly fitted. Your therapist will help you with the fit. Other lymphedema patients may be a reliable resource for a good fitter, or you may find this information at a medical-supply store (see the Resources section at the end of this book). But whomever you consult, make sure first that the person is experienced with lymphedema treatment and knows what the proper fit of a compression garment should be. A good fitter also should treat you with courtesy and attention. If a fitter makes you feel intimidated, or implies that any difficulty fitting the sleeve is your fault, think about finding a new source.

The sleeve may be either custom-measured to your arm or leg or bought over the counter in standard sizes that you will have to try on to make sure of a good fit. Since the garment should be washed daily to keep it as free as possible of dirt, sweat, and germs, it is a good idea to buy two sleeves, or even three, just in case one tears.

If you are dissatisfied with store-bought, over-the-counter compression garments, custom-made garments are available from specialty houses. However, with a custom-made garment, it may take as much as six weeks for the garment to arrive, during which time your limb may become more swollen. To avoid this, ask how you can arrange overnight shipping. This will add to the cost, but it can be worth it. Also, ask about the company's return policy. If the garment seems to fit well at the time you purchase it but later becomes uncomfortable, you will want the option of returning it. So find out first if you can return it after a few days for a full refund. Beware of measure-yourself mail-order compression sleeves. These garments, which generally cannot be returned, are often ill-fitting and, as a result, ineffectual.

Proper fitting of the sleeve cannot be emphasized enough. Some people have difficulty getting the sleeve to fit unless they "prime" the limb with an oil-free skin lotion (Physician's Formula and Oil of Olay have oil-free products that are often recommended). Others find that thoroughly cleansing and drying the limb, without applying a lotion, is the best way to get the sleeve to fit. The technique that is right for you has to be decided by you alone. Most people discover this by trial and error.

Buying a compression garment is not a one-time affair. If you are undergoing pump therapy, manual lymph drainage, or complete decongestive physiotherapy, your arm or leg will be decreasing in size and at some point you will have to be measured for a smaller garment. Even with a good fit, a compression garment's elasticity lasts for only about six months, after which it becomes useless and must be replaced. The prices of compression sleeves vary, depending on where you buy them, but they generally cost in the neighborhood of $100 to $150.

When you have your compression garment fitted, make sure that you avoid sleeves with elasticized wristbands. Ask instead for a garment with a soft border. Although it is not uncommon for people with lower limb lymphedema to experience swelling of the toes, leg garments do not ordinarily include toe compression. However, you can have a toe-compression "glove" customized for this purpose. If there is swelling in your hand, a glove (or gauntlet) may be necessary, and if there is swelling in your shoulder, you may need to have the sleeve custom-fitted with a shoulder cap.

The well-fitting sleeve should be unobtrusive. If it is noticeable, you may feel self-conscious or grow irritated at being asked why you are wearing it. Look for cover-up clothing that is attractive, comfortable, and nonconstricting. As for unwanted questions, it's best to establish a routine answer that addresses the subject with as much, or as little, detail as you wish. For instance, you might say something like, "I have a chronic condition in which my arm swells, and this garment helps keep the swelling down." Or you might prefer to use a little humor: "Oh, this? I wear it with everything because I think it's so attractive—don't you?"

A relatively new addition to the arena of compression garments is the Reid sleeve. This device provides a gentle, graduated pressure by means of a unique soft foam insert. The sleeve slides easily over the affected limb and then a series of adjustable compression bands are fastened. A specially designed gauge, as easy to use as a blood-pressure cuff, assesses the pressure exerted over various parts of the limb to ensure that the compression is consistent. As the swelling subsides, the sleeve can be adjusted to the limb's new size. For more information about the Reid sleeve, you can contact Peninsula Medical (see the Resources section at the end of the book).

Putting on the Compression Garment

The compression sleeve is put on like a sweater, from the wrist to the underarm area. A leg sleeve is put on like a pair of tights. It is best to wear rubber gloves when putting on the sleeve; this gives you a better grip and prevents any tearing from your fingernails.

First, invert the sleeve halfway, starting at the wrist or ankle. Then work it slowly up the arm or leg, smoothing out any wrinkles along the way that might cause irritation. Because of the garment's function—compressing the tissues to drain them of excess fluid—it should not be too easy to get on, but you should be able to put it on by yourself.

Initially, the garment will take some getting used to. Since its strong, uniform compression drives the fluid that has collected in your arm or leg back into your lymphatic system, your limb may initially feel tired or heavy. While the sleeve should fit tightly, it should not cause you any pain or numbness. If you experience either of these sensations, remove the sleeve at once and go back to the therapist for a refitting.

When to Wear the Compression Garment

If your doctor or lymphedema therapist recommends that you wear the sleeve only at night, question this advice. Lymphedema has no respect for the clock or the calendar. Without a sleeve, the arm or leg will get larger as the day progresses. Putting on a fresh sleeve first thing every morning, when your limb is less swollen, must become second nature, like putting on underwear. Some people prefer to have different-sized sleeves for daytime and nighttime use because they find that the degree of pressure that is tolerable during the day is uncomfortable at night. If you are traveling by air or exercising during the day, you may find it helpful to wear a compression garment during the day (except, of course, when you are taking a shower or swimming) and bandages at night.

The compression garment should always be worn during exercise. If you are pregnant and you either have or are at risk of developing lower limb lymphedema, it is important to wear the compression stocking during the entire pregnancy. Throughout the nine months of pregnancy, the body's weight and fluid volume increase, which can tax an already swollen limb. In addition to seeking obstetrical care, you should consult an expert in vascular problems or lymphedema treatment. Because infection is a constant threat to those with lymphedema, a compression sleeve should never be worn on a limb that shows any signs of infection, such as open or irritated sores, redness, warmth, or increased inflammation.

The key concept in using the compression garment is constancy. Many people with lymphedema think it's all right to stop wearing the garment once the swelling has gone down. However, it is all the steps of CDP together that offer long-lasting relief: massage, cleansing, bandaging, *and* compression garments. If the garment is not worn every day, the limb will once again swell—if not immediately, then weeks or months later.

Be an Informed Consumer

One problem that some people encounter stems not from the compression garment itself, but from the supplier. Compression garments are often obtained through what are called durable medical equipment (DME) companies. These are the same companies that supply wheelchairs, bandages, canes, walkers, and other such devices. They operate under guidelines established by the Health Care Finance Administration (HCFA), a governmental agency. The way it is supposed to work is this: A patient goes to his or her doctor, who prescribes a particular piece of equipment; the patient takes this prescription to a DME company, which supplies the needed equipment. The patient is then taught the correct use of the equipment by his or her physician or some other professional recommended by the doctor.

It sounds simple, but, unfortunately, there are some less than scrupulous DME companies out there that will attempt to sell patients unnecessary and costly equipment. For example, if you go to your doctor complaining of increased swelling in an arm or leg, your doctor may prescribe a compression garment and tell you where to purchase it. But when you go to the DME company, a salesperson may try to convert a simple over-the-counter sale into investment in an extremely costly piece of equipment. He or she may tell you that what you "really need" is several bandages, at a cost of several hundred dollars. Or the salesperson may suggest that you require long-term therapy with a sequential compression device—at a cost of up to five thousand dollars. He or she may even contact your physician to have these things prescribed and proceed to instruct you on their use. All this from an unlicensed person with no medical credentials or training in lymphedema therapy! Some DME companies have contracts with hospitals to provide bedside treatment and measurement for garments. Although the HCFA has deemed this an invasion of privacy by nonprofessionals, the practice continues on a daily basis.

The danger here to uninformed patients is obvious. As we have seen, not only can sequential pumps harm the lymphatic system if not used correctly and strictly under the guidance of a doctor, but without comprehensive lymphedema therapy, the condition is apt to grow worse. If you visit a DME company, buy or rent only the equipment your doctor has prescribed. If a DME salesperson tries to sell you additional equipment, ask him or her for literature, take notes, and tell him or her that you will discuss the suggestion with the people who are treating you. You may save yourself a lot of money and a lot of grief.

ELEVATION

"Just about all you can do is keep your arm (or leg) elevated," is the advice that lymphedema sufferers have heard over and over through the years. Translated into plain English, this means, "There's nothing more we can do."

As you have already learned, there is a lot more you can do! But that doesn't mean that you should ignore the advice to elevate your limb. If the limb has not yet developed pitting edema (see page 14), elevation may encourage increased lymph flow, and keeping the arm or leg in a raised position may reduce some of the swelling.[7]

Elevating a limb is fine for those occasions (rare as they may be) that you can find the time to rest on your couch or watch television and prop your arm or leg up on several pillows, or when you go to bed. But it is certainly not the sole solution for this chronic condition, nor should it be. For one thing, it is unrealistic. No one can spend his or her days with a limb in the air—the very thought of such a thing is ridiculous. Moreover, the relief elevation offers is temporary; put the limb down and the fluid flows back into the tissues. Elevation should be considered only one part of a comprehensive plan of action—along with (not instead of) other strategies that may afford you long-lasting relief and comfort.

MEDICATION

People with lymphedema are often prescribed a variety of medications. The most common include diuretics, antibiotics, and steroids. There are also other drugs that are not in wide use for lymphedema—but perhaps should be.

When it comes to medication, everyone—not only people with lymphedema—must be vigilant, asking his or her doctor and pharmacist about the intended effects, side effects, and possible dangers of any drug prescribed. Once you begin taking a medication, you must monitor yourself, paying close attention to any signs of a negative reaction. And you must report any suspected reaction to your doctor immediately. Often, if a medication is effective but causes unpleasant side effects, it need not be abandoned. Sometimes it is simply a matter of waiting it out until your system becomes accustomed to the new medication. Or it may be possible to decrease the dosage, alter the way you take the drug, or add a second medication that acts as an antidote to the side effects of the first. However, you should never make these adjustments on your own. Always consult with your doctor first.

Diuretics

The body may retain water for a variety of reasons. These range from transitory causes such as monthly hormonal fluctuations or hot weather to more complicated conditions such as congestive heart failure or kidney malfunction. This kind of fluid retention is known as ordinary edema. To alleviate the bloating, discomfort, and potential danger of ordinary edema, doctors usually first recommend restricting fluid intake and switching to a low-salt diet. If symptoms remain in spite of these measures, a diuretic—a drug that enhances the ability of the kidneys to excrete fluid—is commonly prescribed.

It would seem logical that a drug that promotes the excretion of fluids would be effective in ridding the body of the accumulation of fluid that results from lymphedema. Unfortunately, this is true only in certain cases. That is because lymphedema involves not only excess fluid, but also accumulations of protein. Diuretics promote the reabsorption of fluid back into the blood vessels, but they cannot remove protein from the tissues and return it to the blood circulation. Only a normally functioning lymphatic system can do that. Hence, diuretics are of limited value, if any at all, in treating lymphedema. In fact, diuretics may mobilize and remove fluid from all parts of the body *except* the lymphedematous limb. Some experts in lymphedema treatment believe that diuretics may even be detrimental to those with the condition.[8]

Nevertheless, doctors do sometimes prescribe diurectics for lymphedema treatment, often because they are unaware of the ineffectiveness of these drugs in treating the condition. On the other hand, if you have both lymphedema and ordinary edema, diuretics may be of some help in alleviating the ordinary edema. It is important to be aware of the possible side effects of these drugs, particularly the side effects associated with the class of diuretics known as thiazides. Commonly prescribed thiazides include chlorothiazide (also sold under the brand name Diuril, among others), hydrochlorothiazide (Esidrix, HydroDiuril, Oretic, and others), and polythiazide. Thiazides can cause the body to excrete too much potassium, and a deficiency of this mineral can lead to muscle weakness and abnormal heart rhythm. It is therefore a good idea to have your potassium level tested before taking a thiazide diuretic. If you are found to be low in potassium, your doctor may recommend that you take a potassium supplement and restrict your sodium intake to 2,000 milligrams a day (a good idea in any case), and also that you avoid the use of laxatives, which can deplete the system of potassium even further. You may be able to maintain a normal potassium level, however, by eating a potassium-rich diet. Good sources of potassium include bananas, orange juice, flounder, potatoes, prunes, dates, and figs. Or you may be interested in natural diuretics (a detailed discussion of these will be found in Chapter 7).

Antibiotics

Antibiotics, which are agents that destroy or inhibit the growth of microorganisms, are not effective against lymphedema itself, but they are often necessary to combat the secondary effects of the condition. They may be used at the first sign of cellulitis or other infections, or if the skin is weeping lymphatic fluid. Oral antibiotics—usually penicillin or erythromycin—are commonly prescribed. If you are allergic to these drugs, your doctor should be able to prescribe an equally effective alternative. At times, it may be necessary to stay on a regimen of medication for weeks, even months, to protect against further infection.

Cellulitis is considered a dermatological emergency. Untreated, it may progress to lymphangitis and/or lymphadenitis (see page 28), and may even be life-threatening. If you develop cellulitis, you must begin taking antibiotics immediately, possibly intravenously.

Like all medications, antibiotics can cause side effects. The most common are digestive upsets and fungal (yeast) infections. Many people find it helpful to eat yogurt as long as they are on antibiotics. If you are prone to developing fungal infections, your doctor may prescribe an antifungal medication such as fluconazole (Diflucan).

Steroids

Steroids are synthetic versions of cortisone, a hormone manufactured by the adrenal glands. They are powerful drugs whose use must be carefully monitored. Steroids also have a depressive effect on the immune system and can cause water retention and mental depression. In addition, their use must be discontinued only over a period of time, not abruptly.

Steroids are used primarily to reduce inflammation. Although not commonly prescribed for lymphedema treatment, they are sometimes utilized if the swelling that occurs is related to enlarged lymph nodes or the obstruction of lymph flow by a tumor.

Benzopyrones

Benzopyrones (also called coumarins) are a group of drugs that have been found to improve chronic lymphedema by helping to remove stagnant protein in tissue spaces. They work by stimulating immune cells called macrophages to break down protein deposits. When these deposits leave the body, less fluid is retained and the edema decreases. In addition, an increased amount of oxygen is able to reach the tissues, thereby enhancing wound healing.

In clinical trials in Australia, France, India, and China, both oral and topical benzopyrones have been found to bring about wide-ranging improvements in lymphedema, including a significant reduction of swelling, improved mobility of the limb, a lessening of pain, and a reduction in the severity of lymphedema attacks—all without the use of a compression garment.[9]

Lymphedema experts Drs. John and Judith Casley-Smith used benzopyrones in the treatment of 600 limbs and found an average reduction in edema of 60 to 90 percent during the four-week course of treatment. Doctors who use these drugs recommend that they be taken orally for three months before comprehensive decongestive therapy begins.

At present, no "safe" dosage of benzopyrones has been established. They appear to be relatively nontoxic if taken in proper amounts. Even when these drugs were taken over a period of months or years, patients (including children) who reported side effects described only mild gastrointestinal symptoms, such as diarrhea or nausea. These digestive discomforts can easily be helped with mild medications or adjustments in diet. However, too-high dosages of benzypyrones can cause major side effects, including liver damage and, possibly, death. In 1997, Australia canceled the registration of a type of benzopyrone sold under the brand name Lodema following the death of a lymphedema patient who took it after cancer treatment.

Despite apparent successes abroad, many professionals who treat lymphedema in this country are skeptical about the safety and/or value of benzopyrones. Both the National Lymphedema Network (NLN) and the National Association of Breast Cancer Organizations (NABCO) strongly advise patients not to take benzopyrones outside of a clinical trial setting. And preliminary findings from a randomized double-blind placebo-controlled clinical trial conducted by the Mayo Clinic in Rochester, Minnesota, found no substantial benefit from benzopyrone treatment.[10] No benzopyrones—whether in tablet, capsule, powder, ointment, or cream form—have been approved for regular prescription use by the FDA. However, there are several benzopyrones that are used clinically by some U.S. doctors. Benzopyrones can be obtained only by a physician's prescription, and are available only at compounding pharmacies—pharmacies that have special permission to prepare compounds. Compounding pharmacies prepare, mix, assemble, package, or label drugs and devices that are not available commercially—in other words, they customize these drugs and devices—according to doctors' specifications to meet individual patients' needs. Pharmacists make the preparations from scratch, using raw chemicals, powders, or devices. There are over 2,000 compounding pharmacies in the United States and Canada, and they dispense approximately 43,000 compounded prescriptions each day. The right to compound is regulated under the pharmacy laws of each of the fifty states. For information about how to find a compounding pharmacy in your area, see the Resources section at the end of the book.

SURGERY

For the most part, surgery for lymphedema is considered a last resort, and surgical options usually are not employed.[11] For one thing, success with surgical approaches to lymphedema has been limited. In addition, the risk of complications is generally high. This is one more area in which research is sorely lacking, and is greatly needed.

In this country and in Europe, some success has been reported in the treatment of early lymphedema cases by anastomosing (connecting) healthy blood vessels to one another to create new lymphatic channels. Other procedures that have been used include microsurgery to create new lymphatic channels and debulking procedures, in which the greatly enlarged tissue beneath the skin is removed. However, these techniques often end up worsening the lymphedema. Some doctors have used liposuction, a procedure in which fat is removed from selected areas, to debulk swollen lymphedematous limbs, but further study is needed to evaluate the usefulness of liposuction in the treatment of lymphedema.[12]

Laser surgery can be used to treat certain skin complications associated with lymphedema. Occasionally, in an area of chronic lymphedema, nodules called lymphangiomas can develop on the skin as a result of the accumulation of stagnant lymphatic fluid in the underlying tissues. These lesions often bleed, ooze, and become infected. The carbon dioxide laser has been used successfully to treat these nodules by vaporizing the skin lesions, as well as partially sealing the lymphatic vessels.[13] Laser therapy can be performed under local anesthesia and can be repeated as needed.

EXPERIMENTAL THERAPY

Another treatment for lymphedema, still in the experimental stage, involves multiple injections of a patient's own lymphocytes (white blood cells) into areas of the body affected by lymphedema. The idea behind this treatment is that lymphocytes produce substances called cytokines, which activate macrophages (see page 61) to digest excess protein, causing the edema to subside. One study showed that this treatment caused a rapid reduction of swelling in lymphedema patients.[14] Additional studies are underway.[15]

TREATMENT FOR COMMON COMPLICATIONS

In addition to seeking treatment for the swelling of lymphedema, people afflicted with this condition often must seek ways to manage its secondary effects. We have already mentioned the use of antibiotics to combat infection and laser surgery to remove lymphangiomas. Two other problems that people with lymphedema may have to deal with are pain and the development of lymphedema ulcers.

Pain

The pain of lymphedema comes about because the skin swells and may even be infected. Although it is usually not intractable, the pain can be chronic and energy-sapping, as well as downright demoralizing at times. Both the severity and type of pain caused by lymphedema vary from person to person, much like any pain. Ask four or ten or one hundred women to describe the pain of childbirth and you will get four or ten or one hundred different descriptions! During a flare-up, many people describe the pain of lymphedema as varying from dull to intense but constant, with the surface of the skin feeling bruised and sensitive. While some people say they experience no pain, others report that their limbs feel chronically heavy. The onset of cellulitis is usually accompanied by severe pain.

Pain is a red-flag warning by which your body tells your brain that something is wrong. Like a fever, it is the body's way of alerting you to pay attention. Sometimes you can analyze the pain yourself and do something about it. Are your shoes too tight? Is your clothing too constricting? Is your environment too warm? Did you inadvertently scratch yourself and cause an inflammation? Are you overtired? (Fatigue can exacerbate the perception of pain.) In these cases, the remedy is simple: Put on looser clothing, seek a cooler room, apply topical antibiotics to the scratch, get some rest. In many cases, over-the-counter painkillers such as aspirin or ibuprofen (Advil, Nuprin, and others) provide relief. If the pain persists despite these measures, by all means consult your doctor.

There are several strategies that can help you manage—or even eliminate—your pain:

• Monitor your pain carefully. When did it start? Where is it located? How long did it last? If you consult your doctor or lymphedema therapist about the pain, this information will help him or her determine the most effective treatment for it.

• If you are wearing a compression garment that is too tight, remove it at once and go back to the therapist for a refitting. These garments should not cause any pain or numbness in your limb.

• Maintain your exercise routine scrupulously (exercise will be discussed in detail in Chapter 7). In addition to stimulating the flow of lymph, exercise stimulates the production of brain chemicals called endorphins that decrease pain and elevate mood.

• If you are having skin problems, do not hesitate to consult a dermatologist who is familiar with lymphedema. He or she may recommend treatments you will be able to continue at home, such as cleansing, applying dry-wound and/or colloidal dressings, and applying topical antibiotic, nonantibiotic, and vitamin ointments.

• Seek out qualified professionals who are knowledgeable about mind-body pain-reducing techniques such as guided imagery, hypnotherapy, acupuncture, biofeedback, and meditation. All of these methods have proven immensely helpful in pain management. (More about these techniques in Chapter 7.)

• Discuss any pain you may be having with your doctor and lymphedema therapist. Although pain can be upsetting, try to remember that once attended to, it can usually be managed or eliminated.

Sometimes, the solution to pain is surprisingly simple; other times, it is more complicated. However, if the source of the pain is diagnosed and aggressive treatment begun, you will be well on your way to making this symptom a thing of the past. Keep heart!

Lymphedema Ulcers

The development of ulcers on an affected limb is a serious and sometimes chronic problem that can occur as a complication of lymphedema. Ulcers are inflamed sores that may lead to localized areas of tissue death. An ulcer can develop if an injury to the tissues goes untreated. The ulcer is then fueled by an inadequate oxygen supply, which results in an insufficient supply of nutrition to the cells and tissues. When tissues are swollen and fibrotic deposits occur, the diffusion of oxygen from the blood into the tissues is impeded and the tissues are literally starved of much-needed repair material.

Lymphedema ulcers require prompt and ongoing treatment by a dermatologist familiar with the condition. While some lymphedema patients have found that applying vitamin E or aloe ointment to their ulcers is helpful, others have had allergic reactions to these agents that resulted in further inflammation and pain. Self-treatment for this very serious condition is not recommended. Treatment may include thorough cleansing with hydrogen peroxide and the topical application of an antibiotic ointment like polysporin, followed by the application of a dry-wound dressing that will not stick to the ulcer. Colloidal dressings, which retain moisture, may be used to prevent the development of a scab that, if picked or scratched, can lead to further inflammation of the area. Some doctors recommend the topical application of zinc oxide, introduced into the tissues via iontophoresis, a process in which an electric current is used to infuse soluble minerals into the tissues, increasing blood flow and providing pain relief.[16]

Once lymphedema is diagnosed, either by your doctor or you, the quest for treatment becomes a compelling priority. It is important to remember that help is out there! By following a few guidelines, you will find the treatment you need, and start on your path to effective management of your condition.

Learn as much as possible about your condition—and share what you learn with your doctor. Seek out credible sources of information, and don't hesitate to double-check what they tell you. Once you start networking with other people to learn about lymphedema, you may hear conflicting information, so it can be valuable to check your sources. When you finally find a lymphedema therapist, don't be shy about asking him or her everything about your treatment. And while there is no cure for lymphedema, be encouraged that, with proper treatment, it can be managed effectively.

4

Alternative Treatments

Alternative medicine, also called complementary or holistic medicine, is just what it sounds like—an alternative to conventional medicine. There are several underlying principles that set alternative medicine apart from mainstream, or allopathic, medicine: a belief in the mind-body connection, a focus on health rather than illness, and an interest in utilizing ancient healing practices.

Over the past few decades, increasing numbers of people have turned to alternative treatment approaches ranging from meditation to hypnotherapy, from shiatsu to reflexology, from aromatherapy to herbalism, from acupuncture to guided imagery—not to mention more esoteric practices such as healing with crystals and other "of-the-earth" elements. Alternative healing is now a multibillion-dollar-a-year industry.

In the early 1990s, the very mainstream National Institutes of Health established an Office of Alternative Medicine (OAM) to explore the ancient and not-so-ancient alternative healing techniques that so many Americans find so appealing. The OAM evaluates these treatments through grants, contracts, fellowships, and cooperative agreements with various research institutions, with an eye to learning which of these treatments are effective and suitable for human use. Some of the subjects on which research is currently underway include Chinese and Indian herbology, acupuncture, electrochemical currents, anti-hepatitis plants, music and dance therapies, antioxidant vitamins, macrobiotic diets, and prayer. By studying these and other potential remedies, scientists hope to find the answers to human ills through diet, nutrition, lifestyle, mind-body control, herbal medicine, and new biological and pharmacological interventions.

Although increasing numbers of medical doctors today employ treatments that ten or twenty years ago would have been considered in a "fringe" category at best, many of those who practice conventional medicine—which actually gained a firm foothold in this country only in the last 100 years—are still skeptical, and sometimes downright contemptuous, of many alternative practices. Without the kind of proof of efficacy that comes from reports of clinical trials in peer-reviewed medical journals, most alternative treatments are unlikely to be recommended by MDs, even if these treatments might, in fact, help patients. It is important to remember that just because an alternative remedy is considered unproven by the medical establishment, that does not necessarily mean it doesn't work. Indeed, millions of people attest to the effectiveness of various "unproven" treatments.

When it comes to lymphedema, we have spoken to many people who are increasingly suspicious of and disaffected with modern medicine. It is ironic that as medicine has made greater and greater advances, our society has seen a proliferation of medical malpractice suits, an increased distrust of doctors, and a greater reliance on therapies that have their origins in another age. One reason for this seems to be that, in our age of specialization, people feel depersonalized, unimportant, and like, in the words of one woman we know, "just another number" in their dealings with the health-care establishment.

There is no longer any serious doubt, either in the medical community or among the lay public, that healing is a multifaceted phenomenon, involving not only the physical self, but also the psychological and spiritual aspects of the human experience—in short, the whole person. The relatively new discipline of psychoneuroimmunology, which focuses on the interplay between the brain, the mind, and the immune system, has demonstrated that the breakdown of health involves quite a bit more than germs and broken bones, and, conversely, that overcoming ill health involves quite a bit more than the art of diagnosis, the administration of drugs, or the skill of surgery.

We are not aware of any claims made by practitioners of the therapies discussed in this chapter that relate specifically to lymphedema. But over and over, people with lymphedema have told us of the successes they have had in alleviating their symptoms and boosting immune function with nontoxic, alternative treatments. If you choose to try any of these strategies, we suggest that you seek the services of someone who is trained, experienced, and licensed in the technique, and also that you use it in addition to, not in place of, conventional treatments.

GUIDED IMAGERY

Guided imagery is a technique in which you help the healing process by visualizing mental pictures and images. O. Carl Simonton, a medical doctor, and Stephanie Simonton, a psychologist, have utilized this technique with great success in the treatment of gravely ill cancer patients.[1] Hypnosis or relaxation training can help you to attain the focus needed to visualize mental pictures and images. Many people also use cassette tapes or soothing background music to help them establish and sustain the pictures in their minds.

In guided imagery, you form in your mind a picture or pictures that represent healing in the most vivid detail possible. For instance, you might establish a mental image of what a lymphatic vessel looks like (an anatomy book might help here). Once you have a mental picture of a lymphatic vessel, picture the damage. Is the vessel pinched, whitish, and limp, or raw and sore? Once these images are vivid, you can go on to invoke any number of other images—this depends on your imagination.

For instance, you may imagine what the different components of your immune system look like. You might imagine the infection-fighting white blood cells as looking like tiny combat soldiers—and then send them into battle, directing them to the damaged vessels to do their work. Or you might imagine the fibrotic deposits that are blocking your lymph flow as looking like corks or boulders—and then imagine them toppling over or breaking down into tiny, absorbable fragments. There is no limit on the use of your imagination, and guided imagery is the perfect place to use it.

There are various types of health-care practitioners—registered nurses, social workers, and psychotherapists, for instance—who may have taken courses in guided imagery and utilize it as part of their treatment. Your doctor or lymphedema therapist may be able to recommend someone who is familiar with this technique. If not, there are organizations that may be able to help, including the Academy for Guided Imagery, the American Holistic Medical Association, the American Holistic Nurses Association, Exceptional Cancer Patients, and the Simonton Cancer Center (see the Resources section at the end of this book).

Many people who have read about this technique in health magazines have tried it on their own with positive results. The key to success with guided imagery is to relax your mind enough to allow vivid mental images to appear and then to spend at least twenty to thirty minutes every day following your imagination's lead. It is best to find a quiet spot to do this, but don't worry about the doorbell or telephone ringing and interrupting your thoughts. You should be aware of outside noises but they will not intrude on your concentration.

Some people find that guided imagery "works" after only one or two sessions. For chronic problems such as lymphedema, however, it may take weeks or even months to realize that you have brought about some desired changes. A number of people have told us that by doing guided imagery they felt better simply because they were actively participating in their own treatment. "When I pictured my immune cells in combat," one woman said, "I felt 'in control' of an out-of-control condition."

HYPNOTHERAPY

In this type of treatment, a hypnotherapist guides you into a state of deep rest that resembles a trance. In this state—which has been described as being more like super-awareness than sleep—you become receptive to the therapist's suggestions. Some studies suggest it is the limbic system in the brain—the seat of emotion—that is stimulated under hypnosis, thus becoming open to suggestions the conscious mind would resist.

When you go to a hypnotherapist, you explain the reason for the visit and what you expect from the therapy. This information guides the therapist in bringing about the desired changes. Although not all people are receptive to hypnosis, those who are have reported success in breaking decades-long habits like smoking, overcoming phobias, and experiencing significant reductions in pain.

If you have lymphedema in an arm, the hypnotherapist's suggestion might involve deep relaxation of the muscles that surround the shoulder, bringing about increased mobility and decreased pain and discomfort. Another suggestion might work on self-image, allowing you to see yourself in a new, optimistic, and life-affirming way. Yet another might involve getting you to deal more assertively—and effectively—with your doctor, lymphedema therapist, or insurance company.

A typical hypnosis session lasts about forty-five minutes. It usually takes several sessions to become familiar with the technique and able to do it on your own, with the help of a tape the hypnotist has prepared. Even if you learn how to practice self-hypnosis, you may prefer to undergo this treatment in a professional hypnotist's office.

The soothing voice of the hypnotist is reassuring and it is often helpful to discuss what has transpired in the session with the practitioner.

Many people associate hypnosis with hocus-pocus trickery. Actually, it is a time-tested and respected method of bringing about desired change. However, as with any professional you consult, it is important that you learn the hypnotist's credentials, the certification he or she has received, and from which organization. Again, many doctors, dentists, psychotherapists, registered nurses, and social workers have studied hypnosis and become certified in its use. If your doctor or lymphedema therapist cannot recommend a competent hypnotherapist, organizations such as the American Institute of Hypnotherapy, the American Society of Clinical Hypnosis, and/or the Society of Clinical and Experimental Hypnosis (see the Resources section at the end of this book) may be able to assist you.

ACUPUNCTURE

This practice originated in China several centuries ago. It involves the insertion of extremely fine needles into the body at specific spots to relieve pain and treat illness. The spots the practitioner chooses fall along lines called meridians, which represent pathways through which the body's vital energy flows. These pathways cannot be seen physically, but they guide the acupuncturist through treatment. The goal is to restore the body's balance, and health, by moving vital energy from places where it is present in excess to other, weaker areas of the body.

The use of needles may seem worrisome—after all, the threat of infection posed by a needle puncture is one reason why injections should never be given into a limb affected by lymphedema. However, in acupuncture treatment, needles are often inserted in areas that are distant from the problem area. For instance, pain in the hand may be dealt with by placing an acupuncture needle or needles behind the ear. In addition, the needles used for acupuncture are much thinner than those used for injections. Standard acupuncture needles are approximately the width of a human hair. We have spoken to some people with lymphedema who say that to avoid the threat of infection that even those fine needles might pose, they receive acupuncture through needles that are designed to be used on infants. The relief they have experienced, they said, was worth the minimal risk these "infant needles" posed. The needles also are disposable. If you are seeking help and have anxiety about the needles being placed in your lymphedematous arm or leg, by all means discuss this concern with your acupuncturist.

Today, many experienced practitioners, including medical doctors, use acupuncture to treat a variety of ills and even to perform surgery. Many acupuncturists in the United States are medical doctors who were trained in China and have an understanding of the human body that goes beyond that which conventional doctors acquire in medical school. We have known people who sought acupuncture—with great success—to relieve the side effects of chemotherapy, to reduce pain, and to help them abandon dangerous habits. We do not know if it is possible for acupuncture to open up lymphatic pathways and break down fibrotic deposits, but it is known that acupuncture stimulates the release of endorphins, brain chemicals that improve mood and decrease the perception of pain. Acupuncture is a worthy avenue of inquiry for any lymphedema patient seeking relief.

Acupuncture should be performed or administered only by a licensed professional who has been trained in the technique. Just as you wouldn't allow an electrician to perform a tonsillectomy, you shouldn't even consider acupuncture by anyone who isn't extensively trained and certified in its use. Twenty-six states and the District of Columbia license acupuncturists. There are also national certification exams administered by professional associations. If you are interested in trying acupuncture, look for a licensed, certified practitioner and ask what his or her experience has been with the technique. If your doctor or lymphedema therapist is unable to supply a referral, organizations such as the American Association of Acupuncture and Oriental Medicine and the National Commission for the Certification of Acupuncturists (see the Resources section at the end of this book) may be able to help.

BIOFEEDBACK

In this technique, you learn to become aware of normally involuntary body functions (such as the beating of your heart or the regulation of body temperature or blood pressure) and learn to control them by conscious effort. You are connected, usually through a small sensor on the hand, to a machine that measures skin temperature. By attaining a state of relaxation (stress cools the skin; relaxation warms it) and visualizing the blood flow that warms your body, you can bring about effective relief from maladies including chronic pain, elevated blood pressure, excessive sweating, irregular heartbeat, migraine headaches, general muscle pain, and Raynaud's disease, a condition in which the fingers become abnormally cold and painful.

An important psychological effect of biofeedback is that it gives you a sense of control. For people with lymphedema, with or without complicating conditions, this can be helpful in learning how to reduce anxiety, increase mobility, and decrease pain.

A biofeedback session usually lasts forty-five minutes. Since the technique involves heightening consciousness of body functions that normally lie outside of our awareness, it often requires weekly sessions for a period of several months. Once you have learned to practice the technique on your own, it is possible to relax muscle tension, reduce anxiety, and relieve various symptoms.

Biofeedback practitioners include psychologists, psychotherapists, registered nurses, social workers, occupational therapists, and physical therapists. Any practitioner you consult should be certified by the Biofeedback Certification Institute of America (see the Resources section at the end of the book).

HERBAL MEDICINE

This ancient—and now modern—practice uses flowers, leaves, stems, and other parts of plants to treat illness and promote health. Herbal medicine is considered alternative today, but it actually was the basis for much of conventional medicine. Most modern drugs were originally derived from plant sources: the active ingredient in aspirin came from the willow tree, digitalis came from the foxglove plant, and morphine from the poppy. Some time-tested remedies have not yet found their way into the conventional pharmacopoeia. Nevertheless, in treating symptoms from premenstrual syndrome to high blood pressure to gastrointestinal problems to cancer, herbal medicine, including teas and topical ointments, has proven highly effective in many cases.

For many of the symptoms of lymphedema—including water retention, skin problems, and mental stress—herbal remedies may offer some relief. Some women have reported that cayenne pepper, for instance, opens up the lymphatic vessels; that some herbal teas, such as those containing juniper berries, goldenrod, cranberry extract, and parsley, decrease water retention; and that herbal skin lotions are particularly helpful in maintaining skin integrity, softness, and moisture content.

If you are interested in learning about herbal medicine, there are numerous books and magazines that offer a wealth of information. And in most communities there are homeopathic doctors, nutritionists, and health-food stores that are great sources of information (see the Resources section at the end of this book). You may also wish to consult a professional herbalist. As with anyone who treats you, it is important to find out what training and credentials an herbal practitioner has had. Many doctors, registered nurses, and physical therapists, as well as many self-educated healers, have taken training in herbology and combine it with conventional treatments. If you consult such a practitioner, ask where he or she was educated and what his or her experience has been in treating lymphedema. Also, be aware that herbal treatments have the potential to cause allergic reactions or to interact with medications in unwanted ways. It is therefore essential that you work closely with your doctor, therapist, and nutritionist before using any herbal preparations.

The American Herbalists Guild (AHG), which was founded in 1989, and the International Institute of Chinese Medicine (IICM), founded in 1984, are nonprofit educational associations that offer extensive courses and degrees in herbology. The AHG has compiled a directory of herbal training programs and provides an herb journal for members. In addition, it offers information about videotapes and audiotapes, plus a comprehensive listing of herbs and their actions.

If your physician or lymphedema therapist cannot provide a referral to a qualified herbalist, you may be able to find an herbalist or natural health practitioner by looking under "Health Providers" in the yellow pages of your local telephone directory, asking the owner of a health-food store (or looking on the store's bulletin board), or contacting an organization such as the American Herbalists Guild, the International Institute of Chinese Medicine, the American Association of Naturopathic Physicians, the American Botanical Council, or the Herb Research Foundation (see the Resources section at the end of this book).

HOMEOPATHY

Homeopathy is a system of healing that is widely practiced in England, France, Greece, and many Latin American countries. In the United States, it is less well known, but is practiced by some medical doctors, osteopaths, and naturopathic physicians, among others. Homeopathy was developed over 100 years ago by Samuel Hahnemann, a German physician. It utilizes remedies that consist of minute amounts of highly diluted natural substances to counteract specific symptoms of illness. This practice is based on the belief that a substance that will cause a particular symptom when taken in large amounts will cure that same symptom if taken in an infinitesimally small amount. The remedies are said to act by stimulating the body's own inherent vital energy to heal itself. Furthermore, the correct remedy is determined not by what we tend to think of as the underlying cause of illness (a cold virus, for example), but by the specific way the person experiences illness, both physically and psychologically.

While critics of homeopathy have petitioned the U.S. Food and Drug Administration to ban sales of homeopathic products, increasing numbers of Americans have subscribed to what they say are its healing powers—to the tune of $200 million dollars in 1995.[2] By and large, homeopathic physicians do not recommend that people abandon conventional treatments and use homeopathic remedies exclusively, but rather that they use homeopathic treatments in conjunction with whatever conventional therapy they are receiving.

There are an estimated 500 medical doctors and 1,000 lay practitioners in the United States who have taken extensive courses to become homeopathic practitioners. While many homeopathic remedies can be purchased over the counter in health-food stores and pharmacies, we recommend that if you are interested in exploring this option, you see a qualified homeopath who has studied the practice and become certified in its use. For a person suffering from a cold or ordinary aches and pains, self-medication may be fine. But for a person with lymphedema, who may have multiple, wide-ranging symptoms, it's better to consult a specialist (in whatever field) who can prescribe a particular regimen based on your particular case, and then monitor your progress. A homeopathic practitioner may be able to prescribe a constitutional remedy that will help boost your immune system, which in turn would help to diminish or eliminate many of lymphedema's uncomfortable symptoms. Organizations such as the the International Foundation for Homeopathy, the National Center for Homeopathy, or Homeopathic Educational Services may be able to help with referrals and other information (see the Resources section at the end of this book).

MEDITATIVE TECHNIQUES

From transcendental meditation to the practices of Zen and yoga, the art of meditation has been known to bring about amazingly positive and salutary changes—physical, mental, psychological, and spiritual. Whether done in a group or by yourself, meditation can influence your mind to bring about changes in your body, help you clarify your thoughts, and help you reach your spiritual center.

There are different approaches to meditation. In *concentrative meditation*, you focus your attention on a particular object or sound to quiet your mind and block out the external environment. In *mindful meditation*, the aim is to open your mind to sensations, thoughts, feelings, and images that you may overlook in ordinary life. In *transcendental meditation (TM)*, you recite a mantra, or repetitive chant, to bring about inner harmony and heightened clarity of mind. Introduced to the public by the Maharishi Mahesh Yogi, TM is meant to be done for twenty minutes once or twice a day. Since 1958, over 4 million people have learned the technique, and over 500 scientific studies have borne out its beneficial effects.

All of these techniques bring about what is popularly known as the "relaxation response," resulting in physiological changes that include a decrease in oxygen consumption, respiratory rate, heart rate, and blood pressure. For the person with lymphedema, meditation can help to alleviate at least some of the physical discomfort and psychological stress that attend the condition. Most people with lymphedema, who are already going for treatments and juggling the demands of family and career, cannot imagine taking on yet another pursuit, or another therapy. Meditation is one form of alternative medicine that can be learned easily and practiced daily in your own home and at your own convenience.

To begin, it is often helpful to seek the assistance of someone who is trained and knowledgeable about the particular technique that interests you. There are thousands of TM and yoga teachers in the United States, as well as teachers of other relaxation techniques such as progressive muscle relaxation. Most have taken formal courses of study in their respective specialties and practice the technique themselves. There are a number of organizations and institutions that may be able to help you learn about and seek instruction in different meditative techniques, among them Mind-Body Health Sciences, Inc., Maharishi International University, the Institute of Noetic Sciences, and the Institute of Transpersonal Psychology (see the Resources section at the end of this book for further information).

IS AN ALTERNATIVE THERAPY FOR YOU?

If you think an alternative treatment will bring about instant relief or a miracle cure, you will be disappointed. Whether mainstream or alternative, treatments take time. Why? Because the body takes time to heal. Effective treatments may hasten the process, but nature designed the human species—exquisitely, to be sure—so that it takes time for all major processes to unfold, including pregnancy, birth, growth, and healing.

Disappointment in a particular therapy is, for the most part, manageable. If one strategy fails, we go on to another. But what if an alternative therapy is harmful? With any treatment—whether mainstream or alternative—the potential danger is that it will do more harm than good. In mainstream medicine, there are some safeguards in place. We can consult a doctor or pharmacist or a book like the *Physician's Desk Reference* for information about medications. We can consult medical consumer organizations to learn which hospital has the highest success rate with open-heart surgery. If need be, we can even sue a doctor who has committed egregious malpractice. But what of alternative practitioners and alternative therapies? What if they do you more harm than good?

Here are some guidelines to follow before consulting an alternative therapist or subscribing to an alternative therapy:

• Read as much as possible about the therapy beforehand. Have any studies been done on this therapy? By whom? Were the results encouraging?

• Learn the qualifications of the practitioner. How long has he or she been in practice? Where and with whom did he or she study? Is he or she certified and/or licensed in this specialty? Are you satisfied with his or her explanation of the therapy? Does he or she have any literature that explains the therapy to you?

• Speak to others who have had the treatment. What was their experience? Have they benefited in any way and, if so, how?

• Once you begin treatment, monitor your own progress, just as you do with your mainstream treatments. If a therapy is causing you discomfort, pain, or any other symptom, report it immediately. Ask what it means, and if the treatment should be discontinued or changed.

• If your alternative practitioner is, for any reason, unsatisfactory, do not hesitate to look for another, just as you would with a medical doctor. Some alternative therapies are covered by insurance, but many are not, so—unlike changing from one medical doctor to another—making a change of alternative practitioners at least does not usually involve a bureaucratic hassle.

• Trust your instincts. Just as you would with any conventional treatment, if you start using a treatment or technique and feel that it's just not right for you, stop. You are the boss of your treatment and you don't have to continue with any regimen you are not comfortable with.

It is not uncommon for people with lymphedema to have multiple health problems. Some conditions—such as congestive heart failure, emphysema, diabetes, and extreme obesity—are serious conditions that require ongoing medical treatment. It is important to realize that treatment for these health problems and your specialized treatment for lymphedema are not mutually exclusive.

Quite the contrary. In almost every case, people with serious medical problems who have used both medical and alternative treatments—along with comprehensive lymphedema treatment—have experienced a lessening of their symptoms, a loss of unwanted body fluid, a reduction in infections, and a return to relatively normal life.

Whether lymphedema patients are utilizing conventional or alternative therapies, their goals are usually clear: "I want to feel better. I want my limb to look better. I want to get back to my old life!" This is the cry of every person who suffers with a swollen and disfigured limb, with a myriad of uncomfortable or painful symptoms, and with a life that has been drastically altered by lymphedema. The good news is that treatment is available. The important thing now is to find the doctor and lymphedema therapist and facility that will give you the treatment you deserve.

5
Who Will Treat
Your Lymphedema?

Perhaps no relationship—outside of marriage—involves as important a choice as that of a doctor. Particularly if you have a serious illness or a chronic condition, the choice of doctor can make the difference between a good outcome and a poor one, both physically and emotionally. The same can be said of specialty therapists and of the facilities in which they practice.

As most people know, a truly beneficial patient-doctor or patient-therapist relationship involves more than impressive credentials or immaculate floors (although these things are important, of course). Americans are becoming increasingly sophisticated health-care consumers—asking questions, offering suggestions, participating more fully in their own treatments, and even changing caretakers if and when they find they are not satisfied with the care they are receiving.

This is not always easy, however, for people with lymphedema, who frequently find medical experts, treatment specialists, and lymphedema facilities few and far between. Yet unpublicized as they are, experts, therapists, and facilities do exist. In this chapter, we will discuss the special problems lymphedema patients have in finding them, and ways to maximize the chances that you will receive the best treatment available.

CHOOSING YOUR DOCTOR

If you are reading this book, you have probably already chosen your primary doctor, and possibly a specialty doctor or doctors as well. You may have made this selection after interviewing several different doctors. Perhaps a doctor was recommended by a friend or another physician. Or you may have chosen your doctor because of his or her reputation in a specialty area, an association with a university-affiliated hospital, or geographic location. The choice of doctor should always be made by you, based on your best judgment, and with a feeling of confidence.

When it comes to lymphedema, your relationship with your doctor is extremely important. We have met and spoken with literally hundreds of people who have said to us something like, "My doctor is wonderful. Anytime anything goes wrong, he (or she) prescribes something for me immediately." The problem with this is that lymphedema is a condition that cries out for *prevention*—for timely warnings about what to do and what not to do before it worsens, and for aggressive and timely treatment and management if it does.

Today, a patient's desire to obtain a second opinion (or even a third opinion) is likely to be accepted, even encouraged, by his or her physician, and most insurance companies cover the cost of such consultations. Even if you trust and respect your doctor completely, there is no harm in getting a second opinion. In fact, there can be much benefit. Most doctors agree that second opinions are good medicine. The point of this kind of shopping around is to find a doctor who is experienced—preferably an expert—in dealing with your condition, and one with whom you feel comfortable. This means feeling not only physically safe, but cared for emotionally and respected intellectually. It is crucial to be able to speak freely with your physician, ask any and all questions that occur to you, and receive helpful answers that you can understand. You have every right to expect that a doctor will be sensitive to your anxieties and respectful of your desire to deal with lymphedema promptly and aggressively.

Finding such a specialist can be a challenge. There is no medical residency training program that offers specific instruction in the prevention or treatment of lymphedema, and no single medication or surgical procedure that is effective for treatment. Only a handful of physicians in the United States specialize in lymphology, and few physiotherapists or massage therapists have adequate training or experience with lymphedema treatment.[1]

When we speak of doctors, we mean not only medical doctors (including physiatrists), but also other types of physicians whose methods have proven helpful in treating lymphedema patients. These include osteopaths and chiropractors, as well as others trained and experienced in administering lymphedema therapy, including occupational and physical therapists and registered nurses.

Types of Professionals to Consider

When our country was founded in 1776, the cradle-to-grave health care of most people was largely a family matter. Healing took place primarily at home, with family members providing special foods and herbal potions, soothing poultices and compresses, and fervent prayers for the afflicted. Comparatively few people availed themselves of the services of doctors, and if they did, those doctors came to them! Childbirth was the domain of midwives, not physicians.

As time went on, the mysterious and frightening phenomenon of sickness came to be seen as something that only doctors, with their equally mysterious training, were equipped to handle. By and large, though, it was not until the twentieth century that average people began to go to doctors routinely for their ills.

It is probable that lymphedema has always existed because people have always been vulnerable to traumatic injuries and birth defects that damage the lymphatic system. But it is only in the past seventy years or so, with the advent of invasive surgery and therapies like chemotherapy and radiation, that lymphedema has become epidemic.

Today, the perception of the primary doctor as having the answer to all ills is changing. Sickness is still frightening, but now a variety of educated practitioners—many of them in specialty practice—are caring for people with conditions that were virtually unknown to the public even fifty years ago. One of these conditions is lymphedema. For the person who fears that his or her primary doctor may not know about this condition or how to treat it, it is important to realize that there is help. There are a number of different types of practitioners who may be familiar with and equipped by their training to treat lymphedema.

Osteopaths

A doctor of osteopathy (OD) is trained to treat diseases not only with drugs and surgery, but with manipulative methods that reflect osteopathy's belief in the interrelatedness of body structure and function, and the conviction that the body has great powers to heal itself. Many people with lymphedema have found osteopathy's focus on the whole person—including great attention to the functioning of the immune system—to be very helpful in alleviating symptoms and in long-term management of the condition.

There are sixteen schools of osteopathy in the United States. Doctors of osteopathic medicine are required to take the Medical College Admissions Test (MCAT) prior to admission. Once accepted, they embark on a program that includes four years of study in the basic medical sciences, 1,000 hours of hands-on training, and the completion of an internship. Like medical doctors, osteopaths must take graduate study for further specialization in surgery, internal medicine, or other disciplines.

Physiatrists

Physiatrists (pronounced fizz-EYE-a-trists) are medical doctors. Physiatry is a growing medical specialty that emphasizes prevention and treatment of disabilities through physical medicine and physical therapies, including care for the primary or secondary effects of serious illnesses such as cancer and AIDS. The physiatrist's goal is to minimize dependence and maximize independence by restoring optimal function in joints and muscles, which can be negatively affected by lymphedema and other chronic conditions.

Over the past decade, physiatrists have utilized the significant improvements that have been made in measuring function, quality of life, and health status. You can locate a physiatrist by asking your doctor for a referral, looking in the Yellow Pages of your local telephone directory, or calling a medical center that has a department of physical rehabilitation.

Chiropractors

These specialists base their practice on the ancient art and science of bone-setting and hands-on healing. Their belief is that misaligned vertebrae cause pressure or irritation to surrounding nerves, resulting in a distortion of nervous-system messages to the tissues. This distortion, in turn, causes other systems that the nervous system controls—including the digestive, respiratory, circulatory, immune, muscular, and excretory systems—to be compromised.

In order to bring about harmony in the system, chiropractors seek to correct the misalignments or dislocations of the spine, and concentrate as well on the nutritional, emotional, and spiritual well-being of the whole person. They do not perform surgery or prescribe drugs. We have spoken to several lymphedema patients who reported that the massage and kinesiology techniques that chiropractors employ have been helpful.

There are seventeen accredited colleges of chiropractic in the

United States. Their graduates are required to pass both state and national board examinations before being licensed to practice. Chiropractors are licensed in all fifty states and their services are covered by Medicare, workers' compensation, and most health-insurance plans.

Asking the Right Questions

People with lymphedema are often unsure about where to turn for treatment, and spend untold hours searching for answers to their questions and solutions for their worsening symptoms. In fact, if you do this kind of research, you may be your doctor's best resource for information about the condition. Yet it may be difficult to introduce new ideas or innovative strategies to your physician. Sometimes even open-minded doctors may be resistant to a layperson's suggestions. And you may fear treading on your doctor's professional turf, or having your information dismissed simply because it is "not in the literature."

Most of the cutting-edge research and effective treatments for lymphedema have originated in European countries. Hence, many American doctors, accustomed to embracing only those protocols that are discussed in their own professional journals, are hesitant to adopt new treatments. Yet the new ideas or treatments you suggest may improve your condition significantly, so now is the time to put any old inhibitions you have aside and speak up.

Just as important as the management strategies that may keep a case of lymphedema under lifelong control are the preventive strategies that may allow a person who has had his or her lymphatic system compromised to minimize the chances of getting lymphedema at all. Whether you currently have lymphedema or are at risk of developing the condition, it is important that you have a relationship in which you can discuss every aspect of lymphedema with your doctor, suggest preventive approaches or treatments you may have read or heard about, and expect to work cooperatively to obtain treatments that are maximally effective.

If you have enjoyed a satisfactory relationship with your doctor, then discussing lymphedema with him or her should be just one more aspect of your ongoing association. If, however, you have been dissatisfied all along, now may be a good time to consider finding a physician with whom you can communicate more openly. Don't forget, lymphedema is a lifelong condition, so you will want a doctor who listens carefully to your concerns, is open to new treatments, and appreciates the full implications of this ailment.

The following are guidelines that will help in your search for the right physician:

• Interview the doctor to get a feel about his or her willingness to communicate and be receptive to your questions about lymphedema. Ask specific questions:

✓ *I am curious about every aspect of my condition. Can I count on you to answer my questions in depth?* Your physician should say yes to this question without hesitation.

✓ *I often read and hear about new treatments for lymphedema, including alternative therapies. What are your feelings about diet, meditation, or any of the other treatments that other people describe as helpful?* You want a doctor who says he or she has an open mind where new and alternative therapies are concerned.

✓ *Will you be willing to consult with a lymphedema therapist about my treatment?* Again, your doctor should respond positively and without hesitation. If you detect that the doctor is irritated by your questions or contemptuous of your suggestions, or if he or she appears eager to end the appointment and move on to the next patient, think seriously about finding another doctor.

• Ask for guidelines on lymphedema prevention or management. Ask the doctor if he or she is familiar with lymphedema and has a good knowledge of the lymphatic system, its functions, and diseases. While the doctor may not have an in-depth knowledge of lymphedema, it is important that he or she have some knowledge of the condition, or at least an interest in learning about it.

• Ask which hospital the doctor is affiliated with. You may choose to travel some distance to a teaching hospital (a hospital affiliated with a medical school), as such hospitals tend to offer more modern equipment and therapies. On the other hand, a convenient location may be a more important consideration, since lymphedema treatment is often time-consuming and tiring, and spending extra time in transit may be just too much for you.

• Ask yourself if you feel comfortable in the doctor's presence and can expect not only physical treatment but emotional support. Emotional well-being is essential for good health in general, and it is absolutely vital if you are undergoing the rigors of lymphedema treatment.

• Assess whether the doctor's staff treats you with concern and respect. If not, discuss your feelings with the staff, or raise the issue with the doctor.

• Learn if, and when, the doctor has telephone hours.

• Determine whether the doctor respects your decision to be involved in all aspects of your treatment.

• If your doctor does not provide lymphedema therapy, ask him or her for a referral to a reputable treatment center. Once you have decided to begin treatment at such a center, ask your doctor to forward all records about your condition, and any other health conditions you may have, to your lymphedema therapist.

• It is easy to forget things when you are under stress. If for any reason you are feeling anxious about discussing these issues with your doctor, think about taking notes or bringing along a small tape recorder. Doctors usually do not object to having their advice recorded (but don't forget to ask permission).

• For your own records, ask your doctor for a copy of all written reports about your condition. If he or she is hesitant to do this, you can make a handwritten copy from your chart (it is your legal right to do so).

• Medical terminology can be daunting, even to the most sophisticated layperson. Don't hesitate to ask your doctor to repeat something, more than once if need be, or to explain what he or she has said in a way that you can understand.

Once you have decided on a professional who is knowledgeable about and trained in the treatment of lymphedema, and whom you feel you can trust and communicate with well, relax and trust your own judgment. You will have done your homework and can feel confident that you have made the right choice. Always remember, though, that your doctor is a human being. Do not idealize him or her to the point that you set yourself up for disappointment. If he or she is not available occasionally, make sure you have alternative resources from whom you are able to get support and answers to your questions. Keep in mind, too, that if a time should ever come when you feel uncomfortable about the relationship, it is your right to change it. Although the transition from one doctor to another may be an inconvenience, it may be necessary if you are to have the relationship you want.

CHOOSING A LYMPHEDEMA THERAPIST

The onset of lymphedema is always upsetting. Often it occurs after you have recovered from an accident or surgery, follow-up treatments have ended, and you have regained some equilibrium and are ready to begin, or have begun, getting back to normal. Then, just when you think you have put your experience behind you, the search for answers begins again, only this time with little to go on. Because there is so little written about lymphedema, you may find yourself feeling all alone, as if only you have this unsightly, painful, and frightening condition.

Well, not only are you not alone, there is help. Increasing numbers of trained lymphedema therapists and lymphedema centers now exist. Many of these centers are staffed by people who have professional training in physical or massage therapy and have received specialty training in lymphedema therapy.

When done properly, lymphedema treatment works, and quickly. Within four weeks, there may be dramatic improvements. After a few months, it is common to hear a patient say, "The therapy saved my life." However, you must keep in mind that the goal of therapy is management, not cure. (If any doctor or therapist tells you he or she can give you 100-percent relief, run!) Once in treatment, you will learn how to manage your condition, what to do if and when flare-ups occur, and how to adapt your lifestyle to avoid or minimize those flare-ups. The trick is to find the right therapist, one with knowledge, experience, and compassion.

Deciding who will administer your treatment is a crucial choice that may have long-term implications. In terms of accessibility, trust, and mutual respect, any lymphedema therapist you choose should meet the same criteria as your primary doctor or medical specialist. And like any other health-care professional you choose, your lymphedema therapist must have the skill to give you the kind of comprehensive treatment that promises long-lasting relief from lymphedema's symptoms. For example, a therapist must know precisely how much pressure to exert and where. Choosing a therapist who is both educated and trained in lymphedema therapy must be your number-one goal as you seek treatment. The best way to locate a qualified therapist is to seek referrals from your doctor and from others whom you consider informed.

There is no guarantee that people claiming to practice lymphedema therapy will follow the comprehensive procedures as meticulously as they should to bring about long-lasting relief. Therefore, if you are seeking lymphedema treatment, it is extremely important to make yourself aware of what this treatment should involve, and then to learn if the practitioner you have chosen is familiar and experienced with the technique and has been specially trained to provide it. Before interviewing prospective lymphedema therapists, review pages 47 through 53 and read as much other material on the subject as you can find to be sure you understand the difference between limited and complete lymphedema treatment. If you go to a therapist who is not versed in complete decongestive physiotherapy, you may end up receiving advice to simply elevate your arm or apply a stretch bandage, rather than undertaking the multifaceted therapy that will bring about significant, long-lasting relief. Worse, you may receive ineffective or damaging massage.

Once you have located a therapist trained and experienced in providing complete decongestive physiotherapy, make an appointment to interview him or her. If possible, visit the therapist in person. If this is not possible, conduct an interview by telephone. The following are some suggested questions to ask:

• *Are you trained and experienced in the kind of complete lymphedema treatment that has proven effective?* Obviously, the answer to this question should be yes.

• *Do you consult with a supervisor or the physician in charge about individual cases?* Experience is essential for a lymphedema therapist. Even for an experienced therapist, however, individual cases sometimes present challenges that are best solved when discussed between the therapist and his or her supervisor.

• *How long will the treatments take, for each session and over time?* Of course, each case is individual, but, in general, treatments should be given four or five times a week for four weeks, and diminish as the size of the limb is reduced and a maintenance regimen begins.

• *What kinds of ongoing management will the treatment require, either by you or by me?* You should expect your therapist to teach you and/or your care partner—the person most involved with your care—the correct ways to exercise, apply bandages, do massage, put on the compression garment, and adjust the garment for maximum effectiveness. In addition, ongoing management may require medications for persistent bacterial or fungal infection. If the therapist is not a medical doctor and so cannot prescribe medications, he or she should be in close contact with your MD about your case.

• *What will the treatment cost?* It is important to discuss finances before treatment begins. In many instances, a therapist will allow you to charge your bill on a credit card so that you can pay it off over time. Or you may be able to work out a payment schedule that is compatible with your resources. Unfortunately, treatment at many lymphedema centers is very expensive, and so, for all practical purposes, available only to those who have the ability to pay, or whose insurance companies cover the treatment. (Chapter 10 and the Resources section at the end of the book offer suggestions that may help if you need financial assistance.)

• *What results can I expect?* The therapist should be able to tell you what research and experience have demonstrated about the outcome of lymphedema treatment. Although each case is individual, the therapist should be able to give you a good idea of how your treatment will progress if properly adhered to.

• *Are you trained to apply compression bandaging and garments?* This is a must for any therapist you choose, since bandaging and compression garments are an intrinsic part of successful lymphedema treatment.

• *Do you offer a variety of compression garments?* Garments differ in fabric, comfort, and cost. For the best fit, the therapist must measure your limb before selecting the garment that is best for you, and then do follow-up measurements to assess the effectiveness of the garment. If a pump is being used, these measurements must be taken above the location where the pump's cuff fits. The best person to help you with the proper fit of your compression garment is your lymphedema therapist or an experienced fitter who has expertise in lymphedema. If possible, ask other people with lymphedema for recommendations. A lymphedema support group can be an excellent place to learn about the garment's proper fit and someone who can help you fit it.

• *Are you able to treat any ulcers and infections that may develop?* This is important because ulcers and infections must be treated immediately to avoid exacerbating the lymphedema. If your therapist is not equipped to treat such problems, he or she should be able to recommend a doctor who specializes in the skin problems of lymphedema. If you consult a physician for such problems, he or she should communicate closely and frequently with your therapist about your case.

• *Will you be the therapist treating me throughout the course of my therapy?* It is not uncommon for two therapists to work together, so having the same therapist treat you all the time should not be a basis on which you decide to begin—or discontinue—treatment. As in all professional-patient relationships, however, it is important that you feel you are being given respect and an adequate amount of time for each treatment. If you relate well to one therapist, but poorly to another, you can request that your treatments be given by the therapist with whom you have "good vibes."

• *Do you use pneumatic pumps?* In conjunction with exercise, wrapping, and compression garments, pumps are often used to reduce the swelling in lymphedematous limbs (see Chapter Three). However, they should be used only by people trained in their operation, and never taken home by the patient for independent use. Misuse of the pump can make lymphedema worse, and may even be dangerous.

• *Will you be available to answer questions over the phone?* Often, questions or anxieties arise that require an answer, but not a visit to the therapist. Most lymphedema therapists have telephone hours each day, but it is a good idea to ask about this before making your selection. It may help you avoid the search for a new therapist or a trip to the emergency room.

• *Are you certified and/or licensed in this specialty?* There are hundreds of fully certified lymphedema therapists in the United States and Canada, and their number is increasing daily. All of them have received training and certification from one or more of a number of experts in the field who teach at the Vodder School or the Academy of Lymphatic Studies, and/or from the Földis in Germany or the Casley-Smith courses in Australia. These certified therapists, who include medical doctors, nurses, physical and occupational therapists, and licensed massage therapists, are recertified every two years. Ask the therapist where he or she studied and learned how to treat lymphedema. Determine if you are satisfied with his or her explanation of the therapy and ask if there is any literature that will explain the therapy to you. Also ask for the names of other patients the therapist has treated so that you can speak with someone who has gone through the treatment you are now considering. Often, hearing a first-person experience from someone who has "been there" is both illuminating and encouraging.[2]

Lymphedema treatment is serious business. Properly administered, it can offer relief from symptoms and the best chance to lead a normal life. No therapist should mind answering the simple and nonthreatening questions we have suggested. In fact, most true professionals welcome the questions of an informed consumer, if for no other reason than that they indicate his or her willingness to participate fully in the treatment regimen.

As with other chronic conditions, your questions about lymphedema will go on and on. As your treatment progresses, you may have other concerns, or you may simply be curious about a particular issue. If the answers you receive to your questions are unsatisfactory, consider seeking help elsewhere. If, however, there are limited resources in your area and you truly have no choice of therapists, then by all means introduce your therapist to what you have learned about lymphedema and lymphedema therapy, and encourage him or her to gain the skills necessary to implement a course of complete decongestive physiotherapy. A practitioner interested in learning manual lymph drainage and other facets of complete decongestive physiotherapy can contact the North American Vodder Association of Lymphatic Therapy and/or the Academy of Lymphatic Studies (see the Resources section at the end of the book).

Some people who specialize in lymphedema therapy are eager to share the wealth of their information and resources with their patients. Others are more secretive, preferring that their patients view the whole process with awe and wonder and consider the therapist irreplaceable. It is useful to remember that it is your right to ask about everything that is on your mind and to expect helpful information.

Though their numbers are growing, there are hardly enough certified lymphedema therapists in this country to fill the demand for their services. Given the approximately 2.5 million people in the United States who have lymphedema and the time-consuming nature of treatment, the far fewer than 1,000 practicing lymphedema therapists are clearly not enough to meet the demand. And the demand is growing. Experts calculate that by the year 2003, at least 7,000 therapists will be needed to meet the needs of this country's lymphedema patients.

Fewer than 1,000 lymphedema therapists were trained in this country in the past decade. Contrast the situation here with that in Germany, where over 8,000 therapists were trained in the same period of time! It would certainly help if the American Medical Association (AMA) publicly recognized the benefits and cost-effectiveness of complete decongestive physiotherapy, and if health-insurance providers routinely covered the cost of this treatment. But so far the AMA has largely remained silent on lymphedema and the treatments that work to alleviate it, and the services of most providers of lymphedema therapy do not qualify for insurance reimbursement. The time has truly come for these organizations to—as Ann Landers would say—"wake up and smell the coffee."

CHOOSING A LYMPHEDEMA FACILITY

If you have been diligent about selecting a doctor and lymphedema therapist, you are well on your way to receiving effective treatment. However, even the most educated, knowledgeable, and compassionate practitioner may not be operating in the best setting or with the most up-to-date equipment. That is why, when you are interviewing doctors and therapists, it is preferable to do so in person. Not only is this the best way to assess whether you feel you connect with that person, it is positively the best way to see the treatment facility.

Just as there are good and not-so-good practitioners, there are good and less-than-ideal facilities. Once the doctor, the therapist, and the facility meet with your approval, you can feel confident that, within weeks, you will start to feel better.

Many qualified lymphedema therapists practice out of their homes, in offices they have adapted for professional use. If you choose such a therapist, make sure he or she answers your questions satisfactorily, and that his or her facility is equipped with the tools and equipment that offer true comprehensive treatment. These should include a shower, a massage table that safely accommodates even the heaviest patient, proper equipment for measuring the limbs, garment-fitting tapes, and materials such as the proper bandages and latex chips that may be placed under the bandages. The therapist should also have the kind of relationship with compression-garment manufacturers that speeds the process of receiving the garments. One woman we know spent two thousand dollars for treatment by a home-based therapist who ordered her a compression garment from Germany. When the garment didn't arrive for over six weeks, the woman's arm swelled up and the therapist refused to treat her again without payment. This incident might have been avoided if the therapist had insisted on overnight delivery, even if it would have added to the cost.

There are a few medical centers in the United States that have units devoted exclusively to lymphedema treatment. There are also establishments that advertise themselves as lymphedema centers. When you are seeking comprehensive lymphedema treatment, you should expect to find an immaculate, well-equipped environment and staff members who treat you with dignity and respect. The place of treatment should be a true therapeutic environment, not a treatment mill where you feel you are on an assembly line.

What to Expect

Once you have chosen a doctor and a lymphedema therapist and decided to enter treatment, you will be undergoing therapy unlike any you may have undergone before. This is intensive treatment that may require four or five days a week of your time at the beginning, as well as a total commitment to follow the suggested regimens diligently at home.

First, you should be given a thorough intake interview that covers your entire physical, psychological, and psychosocial health history. Don't neglect to mention events such as trauma, falls, accidents, infections, or surgery as part of your medical history; these events can explain the onset of lymphedema. Also, no detail of your symptoms is too small to mention. If you experience blotchiness of the skin with occasional blisters, you may actually be having numerous infections. An isolated occasion of genital swelling or swelling above the pubic area may indicate you are at risk for genital lymphedema. Don't minimize or be too embarrassed to mention such symptoms, or your therapist will be unable to take the proper steps in planning and administering a treatment program. In addition, if you have a history of depression, phobias, anxiety, or substance abuse, or if life events or family circumstances have prevented you from seeking treatment before, this information is invaluable in helping your course of treatment.

After taking a comprehensive medical history, the therapist will examine your entire body, not just your swollen arm or leg. Because lymphedema often extends into the breast, chest, shoulder girdle, or, in the case of lower limb lymphedema, the genital area, you will be expected to disrobe completely during this exam, after which you will be draped with sterile sheets to insure a respect for modesty and a secure feeling of privacy. Throughout this process, you should feel that your therapist and other personnel are sensitive to your needs.

For example, they should always knock on the door before entering the treatment room, and they should proceed at a pace that is comfortable for you.

Then the treatment begins, starting with three to four weeks of intensive, comprehensive therapy, including manual lymph drainage; meticulous skin care; application of a stockinette garment, followed by wrapping with gauze or foam-chip padding and low-stretch bandages; twice weekly (or more) measurement of the limb(s); and exercise. This should be followed by the proper measurement for and daily wearing of a compression garment, and regular follow-up visits to monitor your progress. If possible, the same therapist—or two therapists working together—should administer the treatment.

Another thing you should expect is an exploration of your financial circumstances. Professional lymphedema centers and private therapists should work closely with you and your insurance company to make sure that your claims for treatment are honored (this will be discussed in detail in Chapter 10). In too many instances, lymphedema patients are forced to forgo treatment, or settle for less than comprehensive treatment, because they simply cannot afford it. Try to work out a payment plan that allows you to get the treatment you need, and/or bring this issue to your state legislature, your doctor, your hospital, or a lawyer.

The Ideal Environment

Lymphedema centers are not exactly common. While breast-health centers, laser-surgery centers, and sports-medicine centers have proliferated wildly in the last several years—all a result of consumer and medical demand—people with lymphedema have had few places to go. Increasingly, however, as patients and doctors learn more about the condition and the special needs it creates, lymphedema centers are sprouting up across the country. Several that we have visited seem to be ideal in terms of meeting the special needs of lymphedema patients.

In assessing a facility, the first criterion is usually the staff. Of course, you should expect that the staff be well-trained in complete decongestive physiotherapy. That is a given, although it is still wise to ask what their professional status is and whether they have studied the CDP method. But the quality of the staff is not simply a matter of training. At a good facility, the staff will treat you with courtesy, respect for your privacy, regard for the all-important issue of confidentiality, and sensitivity to your feelings.

To be sure, you may not have a choice of facilities. If there is only one place available that offers you the treatment you need, you may have to tolerate the remote behavior that seems to be part and parcel of today's medical "care." But don't be intimidated! You are the consumer. Most lymphedema facilities are staffed by compassionate people who are knowledgeable about the condition and sensitive to those who suffer from it. But if by chance you encounter someone who treats you poorly, speak up! Remind him or her that you are the patient and that you *expect* courtesy, at the very least. If you don't receive it, you can lodge a formal complaint with your county medical society. This is a simple matter of writing up the specifics of your grievance and submitting it to the organization, and it almost always yields results.

The second thing you should look for in a lymphedema center is cleanliness. Any facility that has unvacuumed carpets, dust on the waiting-room tables, and magazines that are yellow with age is not clean. Cleanliness is one of the most important things to people with lymphedema. If you are taking every precaution to cleanse your skin (so it doesn't develop an infection), clean your home (so it doesn't expose you to contaminants), and protect yourself against anything that puts you at risk, the last thing you need is an unclean lymphedema facility.

If you feel that a center is not clean, look diligently for another facility. If you have no choice but to go to a center you feel is not clean, again, speak up. Sometimes things that are obvious to you may not be evident to a clinician who is preoccupied with treatment regimens and research. He or she should appreciate your feedback, as long as it is offered in the spirit of positive criticism.

A third quality to look for is the physical environment. It's always nice when a medical facility is aesthetically pleasing, with attractive pictures on the wall, live plants, and comfortable seating. Just like any other inviting environment, the more pleasant it is, the better you feel in it. But that's a plus. More important is a place that has immaculate treatment rooms and an equally clean shower room(s), and a comprehensive array of state-of-the-art equipment, such as massage tables. The facility should also offer in-depth education as well as monthly or weekly lymphedema support groups, or referrals to such groups.

Finally, since therapy is expensive, it is important that the staff take great pains to work with you to help collect payments from your insurance company. Although these efforts are not always successful, it helps to have the professionals who are providing your care exert their influence on your behalf.

Choosing the proper facility and establishing a relationship at the outset in which questions and answers flow easily between you, your doctor, and your therapist will certainly set the stage for successful treatment.

Part III

Lifestyle Changes

Introduction

Once lymphedema is diagnosed, life, as one patient said, "is never the same again." Every normal behavior, every pursuit, every action once taken for granted—all become challenges in the service of avoiding a flare-up of symptoms.

For the person who has (or who is at risk of developing) lymphedema, the most ordinary activities, from domestic chores to choosing a diet to exercising to traveling—the list goes on—can pose a threat. But with the proper vigilance, many potential threats can be eliminated, while others can be managed successfully. In Part Three, we will examine ways to do just that.

6
Everyday Life and Activities

In ordinary, everyday life, it's easy to forget things. This is because, for most of us, ordinary, everyday life is a juggling act in which we deal with a million and one responsibilities, as well as job and family concerns, all at one time! Sometimes life gets so hurried that we forget many of the important things we do routinely.

How often have you misplaced your car keys, forgotten your best friend's phone number, or come home with a bag of groceries but without the milk that was at the top of your shopping list? If you're like most people, things like this happen often enough to make you shake your head in wonderment or laugh at your own forgetfulness. And most lapses don't have very serious consequences. Your keys turn up, you make the phone call later, you go back to the store for milk. It's irritating, perhaps, but not dire.

But if you have lymphedema, or are at risk of developing it, forgetting some of the rules of self-protection as you go about your everyday activities can be dangerous. If you are at risk for the condition, the simplest activities can transform you from an at-risk person to a person with lymphedema. If you already have lymphedema, the same activities can trigger a flare-up.

This chapter will introduce you to a warning list. These warnings apply to everyone who has or is at risk for lymphedema, regardless of the cause or the part of the body affected. The reason they are so widely applicable is that everyone who has lymphedema has a compromised immune system. The key word here is *system*, because lymphedema is potentially systemic. That is, if you have a lymphedematous limb, your entire immune system must fight any infection, mobilize energy, and combat pain. The part affects the whole.

At the beginning, it's not easy to remember every warning. But as time goes by, your new lifestyle will become familiar to you—in fact, second nature—and you will find yourself following these suggestions automatically, to your everlasting benefit.

PREPARE A SURVIVAL KIT

No home should be without a box of Band-Aids, a bottle of aspirin, a thermometer, and an ice pack. These staples ensure that such everyday problems as cuts, bruises, headaches, and fever can be dealt with immediately. However, if you have lymphedema, these are not enough. Now a more extensive assortment of helpful tools is needed—a "lymphedema survival kit."

You should prepare your survival kit without delay, whether you currently have lymphedema or are at risk for the condition. If you will be undergoing surgery or other treatment, such as radiation therapy, that may result in removal of lymph nodes or damage to the lymphatic system, you should assemble your kit before undergoing the procedure, if possible, so the things you need will be waiting for you when you return home.

The following are items that should be included:

• A filled prescription for an oral antibiotic. Ask your doctor to supply the prescription, and also to instruct you regarding appropriate use of the drug. For example, if you are prone to infections, your doctor may recommend that you take the antibiotic at the first sign of injury, or even take a steady low dose of the drug on a regular basis. Penicillin and erythromycin are the drugs most commonly prescribed for this purpose. If you are allergic to these drugs, discuss alternatives with your doctor.

• Antibacterial ointment. Purchase two tubes: one for your survival kit, another to keep with you at all times. Polysporin and bacitracin are commonly recommended over-the-counter ointments. Neosporin is another alternative, although it contains neomycin, an ingredient to which many people are allergic.

• If you have lymphedema of the leg, an antifungal powder, ointment, or cream to place in your socks, stockings, or shoes every day to help prevent infection.

• Adhesive bandages (Band-Aids) in a variety of shapes and sizes. Purchase enough to keep your medicine cabinet well stocked and a good selection of bandages with you at all times. Recent years have seen a virtual explosion of different varieties of bandages, made of various materials, including types that are waterproof, foam-padded, gel-padded, and antibiotic-coated. Consult your lymphedema therapist about which type is most suitable for you.

- Several well-insulated wrist-high (or higher) oven mitts.

- At least three pairs of rubber gloves.

- A pair of heavy cloth gardening gloves.

- A pair of cotton gloves.

- A pair of fisherman's fillet gloves. These are made of fine, flexible metal mesh and are helpful for avoiding cuts and gashes on the hands. They are available at many sporting-goods stores.

Knowing that you have these items on hand when you need them will give you a greater feeling of security and the knowledge that if something should happen in your home that increases your risk of a flare-up, you will be able to take immediate action to cope with it.

RETHINK YOUR EVERYDAY ACTIVITIES

Think of all the ordinary domestic chores you do every day: dusting, vacuuming, ironing, grocery shopping, cooking dinner, gardening, playing with your children or grandchildren—the list goes on. If you have lymphedema, each of these seemingly harmless activities, if not done with care, may place you in a vulnerable position. Strenuous rubbing and scrubbing, reaching up to put groceries away on a high shelf, or lifting a child onto your lap can strain an affected arm. Gardening exposes you to the risk of being bitten by insects, scratching yourself on a branch or bramble, or having minute particles of dirt enter an opening in your skin. Even activities like finger-painting or evening baths with your children or grandchildren may expose your skin to bacteria.

Some activities are so automatic as to be unconscious. Taking out a heavy pot and placing it on the stove, lifting up a pocketbook, sewing on a button, washing the dishes, and making yourself a cup of coffee or tea are but a few of the everyday actions that you must vow never to do again without the proper precautions. However, with a few adjustments, you should find you can adapt these and others endeavors to your new way of life.

Planning ahead is one strategy. If you know you will be using a heavy pot to cook dinner, ask a family member to place it on the stove in the morning. As for your pocketbook, learn to travel light. Take with you only the things you need—your bandages and tube of antibacterial ointment, money in a money clip, your driver's license, one or two credit cards, a comb, lipstick, a mirror, some tissues, and, if need be, your checkbook. And, of course—at all times!—your warning list and pink wristband (see Chapter 2).

Household Chores

As most women, and increasing numbers of men, know, death and taxes are not the only inevitable things in life. Household chores are inevitable, too. Preparing meal after meal after meal, washing dishes, doing laundry—there is no escaping these daily tasks. But human beings are amazingly inventive when it comes to performing these routine—and often tedious—jobs; they function on "automatic pilot" and within minutes, it seems, the food is steaming hot and ready to eat, the dishes are clean, the underwear is folded.

However, if you have or are at risk for lymphedema, every job you used to do on "automatic pilot" must be approached with renewed awareness. At first, this can be anxiety-producing. "Oops, I poured the coffee (or peeled the cucumber) without a mitt or glove," you may worry. This is why it is helpful to have a list in a handy location—perhaps hung on your refrigerator—to remind you of the precautions you must take. Within weeks, your new behavior will become second nature and your anxiety will abate.

Here are some of the things you need to be careful about. First, if you have upper limb lymphedema:

• When sewing, take great care to avoid pricking a finger on needles or pins. Thimbles are a must!

• Always wear rubber gloves when washing dishes. Exposure to hot water can increase swelling. Rubber gloves serve to insulate the hands from the water's high temperature. Also, dishwater is unclean, and sticking your hands into soapy (or murky) water is dangerous, since you run the risk of poking your hand with a knife or the tine of a fork, or cutting it on broken glass.

• Always wear rubber gloves when using scouring pads. The microscopic fibers these pads contain can be abrasive to the skin, and can even find their way through an opening in the skin.

• Wear white cotton gloves and use a potholder when pouring hot beverages such as coffee or tea. Accidently spilling the hot liquid on your hand can inflame the skin and set off a wider reaction of inflammation in a vulnerable arm.

• Wear oven mitts anytime you are working around a hot stove or oven to insulate yourself from the heat.

• Wear rubber gloves when performing such chores as dusting or cleaning the bathroom to prevent accidental scrapes as well as exposure to bacteria.

• Wear cotton gloves while ironing to protect against accidental burns and insulate against heat.

• Wear fisherman's fillet gloves for slicing and dicing vegetables to avoid accidental cuts and gashes.

• Gardening requires special care. Always wear long sleeves and heavy, protective garden gloves to avoid insect bites, scratches, or direct contact with soil. Protection is necessary even for such seemingly nonthreatening activities as weeding or raking.

If you have lower limb lymphedema:

• When gardening, wear long pants and sturdy, well-fitting shoes.

• Perhaps the thing that we most take for granted is simply getting up and walking around. However, if you have or are at risk for lymphedema of the leg, you must not stand for long periods of time, as this increases the chance of ankle swelling, which can worsen the condition.

• If you experience pain while walking, either slow your pace or stop until the pain subsides.

Try not to be demoralized by this list. Don't forget, all of us are creatures of learning and habit. The things you have been accustomed to doing are things you first learned and then got used to. While they may have become ingrained over the years, they were never etched in stone because the human brain is not made of stone—it is malleable and adaptable.

Now your challenge is to learn to do things in a new way. A good way to relearn things is to use the time-tested strategy of counting to ten. In other words, count to ten before you begin any of those tasks you have done a million times before—making coffee, washing dishes, cleaning, ironing, slicing vegetables, gardening, whatever. A ten-second pause before these activities—and consulting your warning list—will help you remember to take those special precautions.

Shopping

Shopping for clothes, normally a fun activity for many people, can pose a threat to the person with lymphedema. Many articles of clothing have labels and/or tags affixed with staples or pins, and it is easy to scratch yourself while trying on a blouse or sweater, or possibly even just holding it up to look at it. Be aware of this on all shopping expeditions. One woman we spoke with asks a salesperson to cover labels and tags with tape before trying anything on. Once you make your purchases and have the items home, take great care when removing the labels—or ask someone else to do this for you, if possible.

When grocery shopping, if you have upper limb lymphedema, ask for assistance in lifting heavy items or reaching for anything on a high shelf. Limit the number of items you place in each bag so that it can be lifted easily with one hand, and avoid bags with carrying handles, as these may cut into your hands. If there are stores in your area that offer delivery service, consider shopping that way and avoiding the necessity of carrying packages altogether. If you have lower limb lymphedema, be careful around shopping carts—they have sharp edges and corners, and it is easy to nick or bruise your shins on them.

Personal Care

Irritation of the skin is always possible when you are wearing a tight-fitting compression sleeve or stocking garment. But even when you are *not* wearing a compression garment, meticulous skin care is vital, as it helps you to avoid flare-ups of swelling or infection. Anything that touches the skin has the potential either to help it or harm it. The following are some guidelines to follow in caring for your skin:

• One of the greatest feelings of luxury comes when you step into your own hot shower. But beware! Make that water warm—not hot. Exposure to hot water can increase the production of lymph, as well as irritating or inflaming an affected arm or leg. For the same reason, avoid saunas and hot tubs.

• Use a pH-balanced, gentle skin cleanser to wash your skin. Avoid harsh soaps. Any cleanser, cream, fragrance, or other product that comes in contact with your skin should be hypoallergenic.

• After cleansing, and before putting on a sleeve or stocking garment, moisturize the skin with a mild, fragrance-free lotion (some people find this optional).

• Shaving your legs (if you have lower limb lymphedema) or underarms (if you have upper limb lymphedema) with a razor is now strictly taboo. An electric shaver, used gently and with great care, is safer. Avoid using depilatories.

• If you have lymphedema of the arm, avoid commercial deodorants, which often contain harsh ingredients. Instead, use a natural-type deodorant. If your drugstore does not carry natural skin- and body-care products, you can probably find them in a health-food store.

• Avoid using talcum powder, which can be irritating. Use cornstarch instead (but check with your doctor if you are prone to fungal infection).

• If you get professional manicures or pedicures, bring your own emery board. While the health departments of some states now require each nail salon to use different tools for each patron, not all do. Since many implements are reused for several customers, it is safer and cleaner to bring your own. *Never let anyone cut your cuticles.* Apply olive oil to them and gently push them back with a clean towel.

• Avoid getting cuts, burns, insect bites, and scratches. Use insect repellent and wear protective clothing if you are planning to be outdoors.

As you can see, when it comes to managing lymphedema, the trick is to protect yourself against injury and exposure to bacteria, and not to do anything with your affected limb with too great a degree of strain or vigor. That means any motion or activity that exercises the affected limb to the extent that it may cause swelling. Other necessary lifestyle changes involve limiting your exposure to certain types of environments; possibly making some changes in your wardrobe; and maintaining a new level of vigilance concerning your body and its symptoms. These modifications too should soon become second nature.

PROTECT YOURSELF IN HOT WEATHER

One very important precaution for anyone with lymphedema is to avoid going out in hot, humid weather. Even in people who have no problems with circulation, this kind of weather often causes water retention that leads to swollen fingers, hands, and feet. If you have or are at risk for lymphedema, this poses special dangers.

To help avoid weather-related aggravation of your condition, as much as possible, stay in air-conditioned environments when the weather is hot, and avoid direct sunlight. Exposure to the sun can cause the skin to burn, peel, and blister, all of which can exacerbate the symptoms of lymphedema. At the beach and in other outdoor settings, take care to avoid becoming sunburned. Always sit under an umbrella or other shade source and always protect your skin with a sunscreen with a sun protective factor (SPF) of 20 or higher. And cover up with protective clothing. The best protective clothing is made from soft, light-colored, tightly woven cotton. Do not wear a cover-up made of gauze, since this fabric does not filter out the sun's rays.

CHOOSE YOUR WARDROBE WISELY

Vanity has gotten a bad name. Although it is often associated with narcissism and negative values, in fact it can be seen as a sense of feeling good because you look good—a basic (if misunderstood) quality of human nature. Since the beginning of time, both men and women have adorned themselves with the styles of the day, from fig leaves to couturier creations and everything in between.

One of the demoralizing things about lymphedema is the toll it takes not only on your wardrobe but on your self-esteem. When an arm or leg balloons to several times its normal size, the clothes you once chose with care may no longer fit, or they may be constricting. In today's fashion scene, however, there are so many choices that finding an attractive alternative wardrobe should not be a problem. Here are some suggestions for how to choose your new wardrobe wisely:

- If you are used to wearing high heels, put them away for rare special occasions or, better still, replace them with well-fitting low-heeled shoes. The lower the heel, the better.

- Look for shoes that do not have any features that can cause a

The Lymphedema Journal

Today's fast-paced world presents us with demands, responsibilities, and expectations that require nothing less than an encyclopedic memory. When serious illness strikes, two things happen simultaneously: Anxiety diminishes our capacity to absorb and retain information just as we are thrust into an entirely unfamiliar world—almost another planet!—that requires us to learn a great many new things.

Keeping an ongoing diary or journal that serves as a record of your complicated voyage is one way to cope with information overload. Names, addresses, and telephone numbers of doctors and other resource people; relevant phone calls made and received; treatment options; doctor and therapy appointments; the advice you receive; medications you take, their dosages, and your responses to them; your dietary regimen; insurance information; and your personal feelings are all among the items you should include in your journal. Having all of this information written down in one place will give you an on-the-spot memory-jogger. Also, by keeping track of times when you felt particularly good or bad—a support group meeting that gave you a lift, or a medication taken early in the morning that made you feel unwell—you will begin to see patterns you can either avoid or repeat. In addition, just getting your feelings out, whether verbally or in writing, is intrinsically therapeutic. Often, writing things down helps you to clarify your thoughts, remember questions to ask your doctor, or resolve troublesome feelings.

Get a blank notebook, preferably one you can add pages to. If you have already been keeping a written record about a health problem that may be related to your lymphedema (cancer, for instance), you may want simply to start a section for lymphedema. However, keep in mind that while the information about the two conditions may overlap, lymphedema is a separate condition, and has its own body of information.

Allocate the first few pages of your journal for resource people and places for immediate access. Include the names, titles, addresses, zip codes, telephone and fax numbers, e-mail addresses, and affiliations of all the doctors and other practitioners you consult for any aspect of your lymphedema. Also include friends and resource people who have helped you with advice and suggestions. Allocate a separate page or group of pages for each major resource, such as your doctor or lymphedema therapist. On these pages, record what takes place during each visit, including advice, new prescriptions, your reactions to treatment, and the like.

After your resource pages, divide your notebook into sections or categories, preferably with tabs for easy reference. The first category might be your general health history before you got lymphedema (including any major illnesses, accidents, or hospitalizations, including for childbirth). The second category might be any event or incident that may have provoked the onset of lymphedema—surgery; an accident; hospital treatments such as IV infusions, injections, or blood-pressure readings on an affected arm or leg; or anything else you believe could be related. The third category might be a record of how you're feeling, both emotionally and physically. This will help you, your doctor, and your lymphedema therapist keep track of your progress, and may help them to alter your treatment plan, if necessary. Other categories might include compression garments, with the relevant information about manufacturers, how to order, speed of delivery, and price; pumps; diet; lymphedema therapy treatments—the list goes on.

Keep your journal entries concise. A typical journalist's format, which asks the questions Who?, What?, When?, Where?, Why?, and How?—plus an additional item, Me—may be helpful in guiding your entries. Under "Who," include the name of any resource person you speak to (your doctor or therapist, an office staff person, a friend, or anyone else) and his or her title, if any, as well as the name of the person who recommended this resource to you. "What?" is the place for information you want to know. Write down your questions, leaving plenty of room for the answers. For "When?," write the date and time of day you saw or spoke to a resource person, made a relevant telephone call, started a new regimen, or anything else related to your lymphedema and its treatment. "Where?" is the location your experience took place, be it the doctor's office, the treatment center, a laboratory visited for blood or other tests, or your own home. For locations away from home, include directions for how to get there. "Why?" should describe the purpose of your experience—for instance, to keep a doctor or therapist appointment, receive a treatment, contact a compression-garment manufacturer, query your pharmacist, or whatever. "How?" overlaps to some extent with "What?" Here is where you record your resource persons' responses and advice, including directions for exercising, taking medication, putting on a compression garment, or find-

ing your way to an office. You might want to divide your journal entries into rows or columns, answering each question that is pertinent for your subject (although you don't have to answer every question for each subject), as in the following example:

Sample Journal Entry

Who?	Jane Smith, Registered Physical Therapist
What?	Asked her experience and credentials about CDP?
When?	December 18th @ 1:00 p.m.
Where?	Her office on 123 Chapel Street, Withit, NJ 07421, telephone 973-1234
Why?	Swelling in right arm since December 4th. Pain, lack of mobility.
How?	She advised me to start therapy ASAP. She has six years of experience; showed me before and after photos. Made appt. with her for January 20th.
Me	Great visit; Smith relaxed me, made me confident of the treatment working.

Or you may choose to make notes in a kind of shorthand that is understandable to you.

Creating and maintaining a lymphedema notebook should not be a chore or feel like another task that you have to complete each day. If you feel like making entries daily, great! If not, weekly, bimonthly, or whatever else suits you is fine—the point is to give you a record of your own journey through the largely uncharted world of lymphedema treatment, and, as much as possible, to put you in command of it. The journal can also serve to protect you, both medically and legally, as well as reminding you of the positives and negatives in your experience, the better to learn from them. And if you follow the simple format suggested above, you will find it takes no longer than five or ten minutes a day.

problem, such as pointy toes or ankle straps. Avoid ankle boots. Athletic shoes or sandals may be the most comfortable, but be sure not to lace or buckle them too tightly.

• Make sure your socks or stockings are not so tight that they leave an indentation on your leg. Unlike a compression garment, which exerts even pressure up and down the limb, the uneven pressure of tight cuffs or socks can interrupt lymph flow.

• Avoid wearing any clothing that presses against or obstructs the body's lymphatic vessels—in other words, wear loose clothing. This doesn't mean that you have to give up your fashion sense, however. Many shirts, blouses, pants, dresses, and other articles of clothing, while not tight-fitting, have a lot of style.

• Avoid garments with tight elasticized waists, which may cause fluid that is normally found in the body's trunk to be forced upward or downward into the affected limb(s). Remember, any threat to one part of the lymphatic system has the potential to harm the entire system.

• Undergarments also should be somewhat loose. If you are a heavy-breasted woman, consider adding padding (readily available in department and lingerie stores) under your bra straps. When possible, wear a strapless bra or a soft athletic bra.

• If you have lymphedema following mastectomy, wear a light breast prosthesis. Heavy breast forms put a strain on the remaining lymph nodes, especially those above the collarbone.

• Do not wear tight rings or bracelets or put elastic bands around your fingers or wrist. Also, do not pull up blouse or sweater sleeves to the middle of your forearm.

These cautions apply no matter which part of your body is affected, since any serious threat to one part of the lymphatic system is a threat to the entire lymphatic system. But don't be demoralized by all these "don'ts"! They too will become second nature, especially as you find shoes, clothing, and jewelry that are nonconstricting and whose style appeals to you. Try to remember that the reason for doing all these things is that they can help to improve your condition.

TAKE PRECAUTIONS WHEN TRAVELING

In addition to changing the way you do certain things within your home, you must make still other alterations in your normal routine when you venture outside. Something as simple as going into a garden or traveling to the beach now requires the kind of attention and vigilance once reserved for emergencies. Naturally, this is true also for more extensive travel.

Air travel presents special challenges, since changes in cabin pressure, immobility, the stress of travel, and the generally high salt content of airline food can worsen your symptoms. The following are measures designed to minimize your risk of a flare-up when traveling by airplane. Many of them should also be used when you are traveling short distances by car, train, or other means.

• If you have upper limb lymphedema, do not carry heavy luggage or handbags, including shoulder bags. Anything that places pressure on or constricts the lymphatic vessels adds additional stress to your affected limb. Generally, twelve pounds is considered the maximum weight that should be borne.

• Use luggage with wheels, so you can pull it along with little effort. Most luggage stores can install these.

• Always wear a compression sleeve or stocking. For flights of four hours or longer, you may need additional wrapping if you have a severely swollen limb or limbs.

• Ask your airline about salt-free meals. Many will provide special diets if given sufficient notice. If that is not possible, bring your own food, and drink a lot of water when traveling a long distance. (Information about the best type of foods to eat will be found in Chapter 7.)

• Avoid alcoholic drinks, which upset the body's fluid balance.

• If you have lower limb lymphedema, ask to be seated in a location where you can elevate your leg.

• If you are prone to infection after air travel, begin taking your prescribed antibiotic a day before your scheduled flight.

• Get a referral from your doctor or lymphedema therapist for a professional you can see should a problem arise when you are away from home.

Initially, traveling may seem like more trouble than it's worth. Several women we know have told us that when they had to make their special preparations for travel, it reminded them of preparing to take their babies to Grandma's house. "When I thought of the diaper bags, the toys, the formula, the playpen, the car seat, and the million other things I had to do just to travel two blocks," one woman said, "I realized that traveling with lymphedema was much simpler!" Most of the planning involved with travel can be done beforehand. So by all means, don't stay home! If you like to travel or have someplace exciting to go, it's worth the time and preparation to do so.

TREAT SYMPTOMS AGGRESSIVELY

Lymphedema can happen anytime after lymph-node removal, surgery, and/or radiation treatments—even years later. In the case of primary lymphedema, it happens for no known reason. If you know you are at risk for this condition, you can take measures to prevent it from developing, but, unfortunately, even people who do everything right do not always succeed in this.

At other times in your life, you may have had symptoms that you would ignore or take a watch-and-wait attitude about. But once the threat of lymphedema becomes your constant companion, you must address such symptoms without hesitation. The need for vigilance is paramount. If you develop any of the following symptoms, seek medical attention immediately from your doctor or from the emergency room of the nearest hospital:

• Redness in any area of your arm, underarm, or chest (for upper limb lymphedema) or leg or genital area (for lower limb lymphedema).

• Pain or tenderness in any part of the affected limb.

• Warmth to the touch of any area of your arm or underarm (for upper limb lymphedema) or leg (for lower limb lymphedema).

• Blotchiness of the skin in any area of your arm or underarm (for upper limb lymphedema) or leg (for lower limb lymphedema).

• General malaise or a flulike feeling.

• Any elevation of temperature.

• A feeling of achiness or heaviness in the affected limb.

• A strained feeling in the affected limb, such as waking up feeling like you had used it.

In addition, you should carry a tube of antibacterial ointment and a selection of adhesive bandages with you wherever you go. If you should accidentally burn, scratch, or cut yourself, or get an insect bite on an affected or at-risk limb, immediately wash the area well with soap and water, apply a thin, even layer of the ointment, and cover it with an adhesive bandage. You should then consult your physician as soon as possible. If you have a tendency to develop infections, take an oral antibiotic as prescribed by your doctor (see page 102). If you do not have antibiotics with you, do not hesitate to call your doctor immediately or go to the emergency room of the nearest hospital. These measures may prevent a flare-up of lymphedema. Also be alert to such problems as ingrown toenails, fungal infection, or blisters, and check with your doctor immediately should any of them appear.

When it comes to avoiding or managing lymphedema, knowing what to do, what to avoid, and how to respond to symptoms helps to put you in control of your condition.

7

Diet and Exercise

The benefits of a good diet have been known since the beginning of time. Today, however, few medical schools offer comprehensive courses in nutrition, and few doctors ask their patients about their diets until symptoms of illness appear, or until a patient is in the hospital, hooked up to intravenous solutions of fluids and electrolytes. Except in special circumstances, such as pregnancy, vitamin and mineral supplements are rarely prescribed.

The same cannot be said about exercise. The benefits of activity are widely recognized as enhancing both physical and mental health, and exercise is often recommended by health-care professionals. Not only does exercise keep people in good shape, but the expenditure of energy richly oxygenates the body and actually leads to more energy! Other benefits of exercise include fewer physical complaints, greater clarity of mind, and more peaceful sleep.

For people with lymphedema, both a good diet and carefully supervised exercise are of paramount importance. If neither has been a priority for you before, this may be the perfect time to reinvent yourself—to embark on a life in which the goal is not merely the relief of symptoms, but the acquisition of bountiful health.

A BALANCED DIET

Whether or not their doctors recommend dietary supplements, most people believe—and good evidence indicates—that eating a balanced diet, supplemented by certain vitamins and minerals, is the best route to a well-functioning immune system and good health. A low-fat diet that includes protein sources such as lean meats and fish; fresh fruits and vegetables; and beverages such as fruit juices and water is not only doable, but makes for optimal health and weight control.

While food and dieting are just about national obsessions, most people are confused about what a healthy diet really is. And for good reason! Wherever you look, "experts" claim to have the answer, yet many of them disagree with one another. Even the federal government, which as recently as the 1970s scorned the regular use of vitamins and supplements, including antioxidants, now recommends that people include them in their diet.

According to Phyllis Herman, a nutritionist and editor, the typical dietary advice that is offered by American dietitians and doctors is to take the skin off your chicken, avoid fatty foods, drink skim milk, switch from butter to margarine, and use artificial sweeteners to avoid too much sugar. But all this flies in the face of evidence from studies of other cultures in which people do none of these things but enjoy vigorous health and significantly lower rates of cancer and other major illnesses than do Americans.

In a study known as the Seven Countries Study, conducted thirty years ago by Ancel Keys, PhD, of the University of Minnesota School of Public Health, villagers on the Greek island of Crete were found to have a 90-percent lower incidence of heart disease than Americans. Their diet consisted of whole-wheat bread, olive oil, beans, nuts, vegetables, fruits, and small amounts of cheese. They ate fish roughly once a week and meat (in two-ounce portions) about twice a month. They tended to exercise regularly and have strong family ties. Cancer was rare.[1] Over the years, dozens of other studies followed Keys's. In 1991, Drs. Walter Willett and Frank Sacks of the Harvard School of Public Health published an editorial in *The New England Journal of Medicine* endorsing the Mediterranean diet as a model for disease prevention.[2]

Nevertheless, few people pay attention to their diets until they become sick or are just plain fed up with being chronically overweight. The proliferation of fast-food chains doesn't help. Neither does the conflicting advice we receive, much of it from people with impressive degrees and credentials.

What to do? As with other major life decisions, you should learn as much as you can and then trust your own judgment when it comes to selecting the best diet for *you*. Most experts in the field of nutrition recommend adhering to a low-fat diet because, ounce for ounce, fats contain more calories than other types of foods and they are widely thought to be the primary culprits in heart disease and implicated in breast cancer. This applies particularly to saturated fats, found in many cooking oils, butter, and animal fats. In the case of breast cancer, a low-fat diet is recommended because women who eat high-fat diets tend to have greater amounts of the hormone estrogen in their bodies, and estrogen has been found to be a promoter of breast cancer. It is believed that reducing fat intake may prevent an overload of estrogen in the body and therefore reduce the risk of breast cancer.

Nutritional experts usually recommend that no more than 30 percent of the calories in the diet come from fat, and that fat should be monounsaturated or polyunsaturated, not saturated fat. For most people, this means reducing consumption of meat and other animal products and increasing consumption of low-fat foods such as fruits, vegetables, whole-grain products, beans, peas, and pasta. Look for the words *fat-free* rather than *low-fat* on processed foods. Avoid butter and whole-milk dairy products. Olive, canola, and peanut oils are healthy sources of fat—in moderation, of course. Among meats, skinless white-meat chicken and turkey are lowest in fat. Veal is also relatively low. Pork and beef are highest in fat and should be avoided. Ground white-meat chicken or turkey can be substituted for ground beef when making meatballs or hamburger. If you do occasionally eat beef, keep in mind that top and eye round cuts are leanest, and that prime cuts have more fat than choice cuts. And avoid barbecuing, which results in the creation of carcinogens.

It might seem that, since lymphedema involves abnormal accumulations of protein in the tissues, eating a low-protein diet might be a good idea. This is not true, however. In fact, a diet with too little protein leads to weakening of connective tissue, which can actually make the swelling of lymphedema worse. Moreover, protein is essential for healing.

Similarly, many people know that consuming salt can lead to fluid retention, and therefore conclude that eliminating salt from the diet may help lymphedema. A low-salt diet can be helpful for relieving ordinary edema (see page 8), but not the swelling of lymphedema, which involves the accumulation of protein as well as of fluid. Nevertheless, we *do* recommend that you cut down on your salt intake and avoid using salt in cooking, because any fluid retention places an extra strain on the circulatory system, and people with lymphedema already suffer from the effects of compromised circulation.

In addition to adequate amounts of protein and limited amounts of healthy fats, a good diet includes complex carbohydrates (whole grains, pasta, and legumes) for energy, and plenty of fruits and vegetables to supply vitamins and minerals—four or five servings a day, if possible. A good rule of thumb is to eat three or four meals a day that contain a balance of protein, carbohydrates, and healthy fats; drink six to eight glasses of water a day (unless you are on a fluid-restricted diet); and fill up on foods high in fiber. High-fiber foods include fresh (preferably raw) vegetables, bran, whole grains, legumes, and some fruits (apples, bananas, berries, figs, dates, cherries, kiwi fruit, papaya, and pears).

Few lymphedema experts have studied dietary regimens specifically for people with lymphedema. One who has is Arlette Dinclaux, a health and nutrition expert. She has investigated the medicinal and other benefits of various foods for people with edema and lymphedema; antiviral compounds that are derived from plants (such as goldenseal); food sources of vitamins and minerals (including selenium, which is thought to be important in lymphedema treatment); and the do's and don'ts of diet and nutrition for people with these conditions. In her book *Nutritherapy for Lymphedema* (E.S.O.P. Publishing, 1995), she advises readers that to purify the system, 80 percent of the diet should consist of alkaline-forming foods. These include apples, cantaloupes, cherries, and figs; asparagus, carrots, cauliflower, and potatoes; cultured dairy products such as buttermilk and yogurt; grains such as millet and corn; and herbal teas, honey, and almonds. Acid-forming foods, which should make up only 20 percent of the diet, include citrus fruits; all meats, fish, and poultry; alcoholic beverages; coffee; lentils; onions; oats; and all breads.[3]

IMPORTANT NUTRIENTS

For good health, the body needs a proper balance of all nutrients—the macronutrients (protein, carbohydrates, and fat) and micronutrients (vitamins and minerals). However, there are certain nutrients that deserve special attention, especially for people with lymphedema.

One group of nutrients that has been getting widespread attention in recent years are the antioxidants, including beta-carotene (a precursor of vitamin A), vitamins E and C, and the mineral selenium. Increasingly, doctors are prescribing antioxidant supplements for their patients, and are even taking them themselves. Antioxidants are helpful to people with lymphedema because they give the already compromised immune system additional help in combating toxins. These nutrients also fight cancer and may slow the aging

Natural Diuretics

Increasingly, people are turning to natural and nutritional remedies to maintain health or alleviate various symptoms, including water retention. The B-vitamin complex, vitamin B_6, and vitamin C are considered by many to be effective natural diuretics. There are also certain foods and herbs that are known to have a diuretic effect. Many of the foods listed here are rich in nutrients as well.[1]

Foods that Are Natural Diuretics

Asparagus	Eggplant	Peas
Bamboo shoots	Grapes	Pineapple
Barley	Kidney beans	Plums
Black beans	Lettuce	Potatoes
Broccoli	Mangoes	Snow peas
Cabbage	Melon	Soybean sprouts
Cantaloupe	Millet	Soybeans
Carrots	Mulberries	Spinach
Celery	Mung beans	Squash
Chestnuts	Mustard	Star fruit
Chinese cabbage	Mustard greens	Water chestnuts
Coconut	Onions	Watercress
Corn	Peanuts	Watermelon
Cucumber	Pears	Wheat
Dandelion greens		

Herbs That Are Natural Diuretics

Alfalfa	Garlic	Parsley
Buchu	Horsetail	Pau d'arco
Celery	Juniper berries	Pumpkin
Cornsilk	Marshmallow	Sarsaparilla
Dandelion	Nettle	Uva ursi

A word of caution: Herbs with diuretic action can deplete the body of potassium. Certain foods, including bananas, orange juice, flounder, potatoes, prunes, dates, and figs help to replenish this essential mineral. The herbs cayenne and kelp also help to supply nutrients lost through diuresis. We strongly recommend that you seek the advice of a licensed nutritionist if you are interested in using diet and nutritional supplements as an approach to managing your lymphedema, and that your nutritionist work closely with your medical doctor and lymphedema therapist to help you.

process by neutralizing DNA-damaging free radicals, dangerous molecules that form as a result of exposure to toxins and as byproducts of the body's normal metabolic processes.

Beta-carotene is the plant form of vitamin A, and the body converts it into vitamin A as needed. It can be found in fruits and vegetables, especially those that are yellow or orange in color. Vegetables rich in beta-carotene include carrots, sweet potatoes, corn, peppers, squash, soybeans, peas, black-eyed peas, and greens (turnip greens, romaine lettuce, endive, kale, spinach, and beet greens). Fruit sources include apricots (fresh and dried), cantaloupe, honeydew, nectarines, mangoes, papaya, peaches, and prunes. Be warned, however, that fruits are also a source of sugar.

Vitamin C—and bioflavonoids, compounds that work with vitamin C—is important for healing and the formation of collagen, a protein responsible for maintaining the integrity and elasticity of the skin and underlying tissue. This vitamin is available in citrus fruits (oranges, grapefruits, lemons, and tangerines), berries (strawberries, blackberries, raspberries, and currants), guava, mangoes, tomatoes, and kiwi fruit. Vegetable sources include potatoes (with the skin), green peppers, turnips, parsnips, asparagus, artichokes, and greens (okra, kale, collards, and kohlrabi). These foods supply the greatest amount of vitamin C if eaten raw, as cooking can destroy this vitamin.

Vitamin E keeps cell walls healthy. It is found in vegetable oils, wheat germ, dark green leafy vegetables, eggs, and legumes. Cruciferous vegetables, including broccoli, red and green cabbage, cauliflower, and Brussels sprouts, have gained a reputation among many researchers as health-promoters and cancer-fighters.

It is known that vitamins B_6 and B_{12}, as well as vitamin C, are essential for optimal cellular function and protein synthesis—both important concerns for people with lymphedema. Zinc is necessary for tissue regeneration and immune function, and iron is essential for the formation of hemoglobin, which carries oxygen in the bloodstream and transports it to the tissues.[4]

Ideally, a balanced diet should supply all the nutrients we need. And by and large, it is best to obtain nutritients from foods, not supplements. Foods contain natural forms of vitamins, minerals, and other nutrients, whereas supplements often contain synthetic forms, as well as additives and sugar. In addition, foods contain many other valuable compounds, such as phtytochemicals, that we are only beginning to identify and that supplements lack. Yet increasing numbers of people believe that our foods have been robbed of their full nutritional benefit by being grown in poor soil and then overprocessed. They seek supplements to compensate for the deficit.

If you choose to take supplements, read labels carefully: The fewer additives, the better. And additives are not the only thing to watch for. Taking too much of certain supplements (zinc or iron, for instance) can have paradoxical or harmful effects. Vitamins such as A and D may be toxic in high doses. While supplements can be beneficial in many instances, they are not always helpful. It is best to consult a nutritionist to help you determine which supplements will benefit you and the correct amounts to take. Many nutritionists will request copies of your blood test results and/or take hair samples for this purpose.

A nutritionist can also advise you as to how and when to take any supplements—with meals, between meals, before bed, or whatever—and when it would be a good idea to stop taking them. For instance, vitamin C compromises the action of some antibiotics. Folic acid can block the effect of methotrexate (Rheumatrex), a drug used for cancer chemotherapy. If you are undergoing radiation therapy, certain nutrients may interfere with the ability of radiation to kill cancer cells.[5] Always remember that supplemental nutrients should be taken in safe and appropriate dosages. If you are unsure about any quantity, don't guess. Ask an expert.

THINGS TO AVOID

High on anyone's list of health recommendations are "Don't drink," and "Don't smoke." Well, here they are again, with reasons that apply specifically to lymphedema.

Alcohol upsets the body's chemistry and fluid balance, and reduces the body's utilization of important nutrients. If you are accustomed to having a glass of wine with your dinner each evening, this is probably too small an amount of alcohol to have a adverse effect. However, if your drinking goes beyond this, now is the time to cut back or stop. If you find this difficult, you may want to seek help. One way to assess whether your drinking has become problematic is to answer the following set of questions:

• Have you ever decided to stop drinking for a week or so, but lasted for only a couple of days?

• Do you wish people would mind their own business about your drinking and stop telling you what to do?

• Have you ever switched from one kind of drink to another in the hope that this would keep you from getting drunk?

• Have you had to have an eye-opener upon awakening during the past year?

• Do you envy people who can drink without getting into trouble?

• Have you had problems connected with drinking during the past year?

• Has your drinking caused trouble at home?

• Do you ever try to get "extra" drinks at a party because you do not get enough?

• Do you tell yourself you can stop drinking any time you want to, even though you keep getting drunk when you don't mean to?

• Have you missed days of work or school because of drinking?

• Do you have blackouts—hours or days you can't remember?

• Have you ever felt that your life would be better if you did not drink?

According to Alcoholics Anonymous (AA), if you answer yes to four or more of these questions, you are probably in trouble with alcohol and might benefit from going to their meetings. AA has helped millions of people stop drinking. Women for Sobriety is another valuable organization that can help. Both of these groups are listed in the telephone directory. In addition, acupuncture and hypnotherapy have helped many people to change unwanted behavior patterns.

The dangers of smoking are well known; it increases the likelihood of lung cancer, emphysema, and heart disease. In addition to these dangers, smoking causes the blood vessels throughout the body to become constricted, and any strain on the circulatory system is dangerous to the person with lymphedema. There are a variety of approaches that can help smokers quit, including acupuncture, hypnotherapy, and stop-smoking groups, among others. A good source of information about the different approaches available is *No If's, And's or Butts, The Smoker's Guide to Quitting,* by Harlan Krumholz and Robert Phillips (Avery Publishing Group, 1993).

Another questionable substance is caffeine. While caffeine may seem to be an effective diuretic—coffee really seems to "get those kidneys going," as one woman we know says of her morning, afternoon, and evening quaff—it can deplete the body of much-needed vitamins and minerals, so we recommend avoiding it.

SPECIAL DIETS

Many people with serious medical conditions have changed their eating habits to embrace special dietary regimens. These include diets that are dairy-free, chemical-free, vegetarian, macrobiotic, or otherwise different from the average American's way of eating. As you embark on the significant lifestyle changes required to manage lymphedema, you too may want to explore new ways of eating. Many people have reported that when they threw out their old dietary habits, they started to feel better, have more energy, and enjoy more robust health than ever before. Here is a look at some dietary regimens people have found helpful.

A dairy-free diet may appeal to you if you have protein allergies or a lactose intolerance, if you believe that dairy products are not good for you, or if you simply do not like dairy products. Dairy foods can be eliminated from the diet without sacrificing the nutrients they contain, specifically, protein and calcium. You can get protein from lean meat or fish or, if you are a vegetarian, from legumes and grains. Good sources of calcium include broccoli, farina, figs, molasses, rhubarb, salmon, sardines, sesame seeds, spinach, and tofu.

A chemical-free diet, also known as an organic diet, consists of foods produced without the use of any pesticides, hormones, preservatives, colorings, or any of the other "enhancements" with which many modern foods are delivered to the market. Since pesticides have been linked to a variety of human ills, from allergies to cancer, many people now seek organically grown (or raised) products to minimize their exposure to these compounds. Organically raised chickens and cattle are raised on natural feeds; organic vegetables, fruits, and grains are grown on farms that use only natural fertilizers and no pesticides, fungicides, ripening agents, or other chemicals. Many supermarkets now feature organic-food sections, as do health-food stores.

The word *vegetarian* comes from the Latin word *vegetus*, meaning "whole," "sound," "fresh," or "lively." There are different approaches to vegetarianism. Some vegetarians, termed lacto-ovo vegetarians, eat no meat, fish, or fowl, but include dairy products and eggs in their diets. Lacto vegetarians consume dairy products but not eggs. Total vegetarians, or vegans, eat no animal products whatsoever. Many vegetarians also avoid refined, processed foods. Regardless of the approach, the plant foods vegetarians eat are loaded with nutrients, including protein, iron, and calcium. Believing that no one food source is nutritionally complete by itself, vegetarians base their diets on a variety of grains, vegetables, legumes, nuts, seeds, and fruits. A vegetarian diet is high in fiber and low in saturated fat and cholesterol.

Although there is somewhat less protein in a vegetarian diet than in a nonvegetarian one, vegetarians believe this to be advantageous. They say that the consumption of excessive amounts of protein has been linked to heart disease, strokes, various types of cancer, kidney stones, osteoporosis, and adult-onset diabetes. Vegetarians get their iron and calcium from dark green vegetables, soy products and legumes, whole grains, dried fruits, nuts, and seeds. Adding foods rich in vitamin C, such as fruits and greens, enhances iron absorption. Zinc is found in whole grains and and whole-grain products, wheat germ, tofu, tempeh, miso, legumes, sprouts, nuts, and seeds, as well as in eggs and dairy products. All other vitamins and minerals, as well as healthy fats and carbohydrates, are widely found in the plant kingdom, with the exception of vitamin B_{12}, which may be taken in supplement form.

Macrobiotics, which means "larger life study," is a comprehensive belief system based on the idea of living in harmony with nature. The term *makrobios* was used by Hippocrates, the ancient Greek physician known as the "Father of Medicine," to describe a way of living for health and longevity. This way of life seeks to restore or preserve health by embracing biological, physiological, emotional, psychological, social, and spiritual concerns.

The primary foods in the macrobiotic diet are whole-grain cereals, supplemented by soy products, vegetables, sea vegetables, fruit, nuts, seeds, and a small amount of animal produce. Fruits, vegetables, nuts, and seeds (preferably locally produced) are eaten in season. People in temperate climates may add moderate amounts of white fish and shellfish to the diet as well. Foods containing high levels of fat or sugar, or chemical additives, are avoided, and the intake of liquids is limited, especially with meals. This is a very disciplined diet. However, its followers claim it brings about constant high levels of physical energy; the ability to fall asleep easily and wake up totally refreshed after a few hours; a hearty appetite for simple, nourishing food and for sex; a positive and happy frame of mind; a good memory; and a profound gratitude for the gift of life.

EXERCISE

If you are accustomed to regular, vigorous exercise, you will have to make an adjustment to this routine if you contract lymphedema or if you become at risk for the condition. Ancient wisdom promoted moderation in all things. If you have lymphedema, this philosophy must now become the rule. However, that does not mean abandoning exercise altogether. In fact, if you have never exercised before, now is the time to start taking that daily walk or spending fifteen minutes a day on a stationary bicycle. The right kind of physical activity helps stimulate the flow of lymphatic fluid and helps to keep you in good shape generally.

If you have lower limb lymphedema and your leg is greatly swollen, walking may be uncomfortable. If you are able to walk without discomfort or pain, however, a daily walk of twenty minutes, either on a treadmill or outdoors, is good exercise that will stimulate your circulatory system and improve your general well-being. In fact, lymphatic fluid moves as the body moves; muscle contractions serve as a pumping force that can facilitate lymphatic flow. If at any time your limb responds with increased edema or pain, decrease the intensity of the exercise.

In addition to walking and bicycling, swimming is a beneficial form of exercise. When you are in chest-high water, your body weight is reduced by about ninety percent, which relieves the weight in your limbs. Water exercise enhances muscle tone and strength as well. Other good exercise choices for people with lymphedema include low-impact aerobics, yoga, and tai chi.

Initially, it is a good idea to ask the guidance of your doctor or lymphedema therapist in developing your exercise regimen. Any program you undertake should be tailored to your particular needs, capabilities, and physical health. There are very few studies that compare the value of different types of exercise for lymphedema patients. Those that do exist offer contradictory advice. However, a number of experienced lymphedema therapists agree that no one knows better than the lymphedema patient him- or herself what "good" exercise involves. Good exercise, they say, is physical activity that feels good. Some people who have lymphedema of the arm are golf enthusiasts. This is fine, as long as there is no discomfort, pain, or pressure. Some people who have lymphedema of the leg are joggers. That's fine too, unless it starts not to feel fine. In other words, do what you can, within reason. But whatever type of exercise you choose, if the affected limb hurts or begins to feel strained, or if you fear something you are doing may worsen your symptoms, STOP! If you have any doubts, discuss your exercise routine and the sensations you are experiencing with your doctor and lyphedema therapist.

In addition to aerobic exercise such as walking, people with lymphedema often perform specialized exercise routines suggested by their lymphedema therapists. These exercises are an important part of a comprehensive program to deal with the discomfort, debility, and depression caused by lymphedema. They help to reduce swelling and promote lymphatic drainage, as well as helping to keep you in good shape. Lymphedema exercises are done once or twice a day for twenty to thirty minutes at a time, with the affected limb bandaged and a compression garment worn.

People with lymphedema usually experience feelings of tightness and a decrease in the range of motion of the affected limb. Moderate stretching, flexibility, and muscle-strengthening exercises, done regularly, can do the following:

• Relax your muscles.

• Increase your range of motion.

• Promote muscle-pumping action that mobilizes stagnant fluid, stimulates the flow of lymph through the lymphatic vessels, and increases the level of oxygen throughout the body, resulting in the delivery of more nutrients to the cells.

• Help keep your weight down.

• Improve cardiovascular function.

• Stimulate the flow of endorphins, brain chemicals that decrease pain and elevate mood.

Each therapist has his or her own routine, but generally the exercises follow a pattern that includes relaxation; flexion of the limbs, elbows, knees, and fingers; head and shoulder rotations; arm and leg maneuvers; massage; sit-ups; and breathing exercises. The breathing exercises are important because they oxygenate the body and encourage better circulation, and also bring about deep relaxation.

Similar to prepared-childbirth breathing, they involve inhaling deeply, holding the breath for a few seconds, then exhaling slowly. When properly done, these exercises promote the drainage of lymphatic fluid. But if they are done improperly, they can actually do more harm than good. This is why you must find a therapist who is trained in lymphedema exercises.

For all lymphedema patients, a twice-daily program of moderate exercise can be immensely helpful, both physically and psychologically. The specialized exercises offered by a lymphedema therapist can be done at home, every day, for years and years and years. Since you will be doing these exercises at home, ask your therapist for printed material, preferably with drawings, that shows you exactly what to do and for how long. Once your lymphedema is under control, you may cut your exercise time down to ten minutes instead of twenty or thirty. But most people find these exercises so easy, pleasurable, and beneficial that they continue doing them, as one woman told us, "just for the fun of it."

It is important to wear a compression garment during all physical activity. Unlike the blood, which is pumped through the circulatory system by the heart, lymph has no organ to pump it. Rather, lymphatic fluid is pushed through the vessels by the contractions of skeletal muscles, and wearing the sleeve while exercising causes those muscles to act as a pump. If you engage in more strenuous exercise, such as weight-lifting, it may be necessary to wear a complex bandage, with additional wrapping that provides more pressure on the affected limb and acts as an even stronger pump. Generally, though, more limited exercise is recommended to avoid taxing an affected limb and risking injury and further inflammation.

If your exercise sessions are supervised by a lymphedema therapist—as they should be—your workouts can be modified as your mobility and strength increase, always taking into consideration your physical ability, your ability to perform everyday tasks, and your social and/or occupational situation. If you work out at a gym, particularly if you lift weights, it is important to get your doctor's approval to resume your regular regimen after lymph-node removal.

There are some circumstances that make exercise impossible. An inability to walk is an obvious example. More common is the development of ulcers on the affected limb, a serious and sometimes chronic problem. If you are unable to walk or have developed ulcers, you may be able to do muscle-strengthening and flexing exercises such as squeezing a rolled-up sock with your fingers, rolling your neck in a circular motion, curling your toes, and flexing your fingers by first making a fist, then extending your fingers. Such exercises should be done only under the guidance of a knowledgeable therapist, however.

For people with lymphedema, the magical thing about eating well and engaging in supervised exercise is the feeling of well-being these measures produce. Simply, what you put into your body affects how you feel and how well your body—including your all-important immune system—functions. A healthy diet can have a positive influence on your entire body. And when you direct your body to engage in intelligent—that is, not too strenuous—exercise, including the more meditative breathing exercises, you inevitably find your energy increasing, your nervous system more peaceful, and your thinking more clear than ever.

Part IV

Dealing With Yourself and Others

Introduction

Catastrophic health problems such as cancer, traumatic injury, or devastating infection leave inevitable scars. These may be physical—a missing limb or breast, scar tissue, a limp, or ongoing pain—or emotional—a lifelong feeling of vulnerability, or fear of follow-up checkups and tests. Whatever their nature, these scars serve as a constant reminder to the survivor of his or her ordeal.

Lymphedema too leaves its scars. One particularly devastating thing about lymphedema is that it often occurs after treatment for another serious medical problem has ended. Just when you think, "Whew, it's over. Now I can get back to my 'normal' life," you find yourself with an often debilitating and disfiguring condition, and an inventory of restrictions that can be more difficult to accept than the condition itself.

The precautions you must now take every day are not easy, to say the least. The most mundane, routine things—paper cuts, a burn from the oven or the iron, insect bites, sunbathing; the list goes on—now become real risks. It is not long before the gravity of the condition sinks in: This is for life! In fact, many lymphedema sufferers describe their condition as a "life sentence." They feel blindsided, afflicted with a condition they were never warned about—possibly never even heard of—and that, they discover, has no cure and few effective treatments.

In the privacy of your home, and in your relationships with people who are supportive, all things can be negotiated. Or can they? Often, the lymphedema patient finds that even among family and friends, problems arise. In Part Four, you will learn that these issues, too, can be dealt with effectively.

8
Family, Friends, and Coworkers

Dealing with friends and family members, no matter how well intentioned, can be taxing to the person who feels he or she must always put on the best face or who is unaccustomed to being on the receiving end of attention and caretaking. For women, who are often used to taking care of others, it can be difficult to be forced to switch roles; for men, it is often hard to accept feeling needy or dependent on others.

People who undergo major surgery or serious illness, especially those who have lost a part of their body or their natural vigor, inevitably go through a period of grieving. A similar reaction happens with lymphedema. Losing the mobility, shape, or normal functioning of an arm or leg, or having to rearrange every facet of normal life, can be devastating.

Even people who face this condition surrounded by people they love, and who love them, can experience feelings of isolation. Often, it feels like it's just you and the condition—the two of you against the world. With something like cancer, these feelings are a reaction to a disease that is openly recognized, talked about, publicized, and part of everyone's vocabulary. The same can be said about a traumatic accident or almost any type of surgery.

But lymphedema is a condition few people are familiar with. Even those most at risk of developing the condition are rarely told about it. As a result, when an arm or leg suddenly becomes swollen, it is easy to feel as if you are all alone, plagued by disturbing symptoms that no one else you know has experienced. In fact, when you mention your diagnosis to other people, one of the most common reactions you encounter is, "Lymphe-what?" Given this general lack of awareness, it is not hard to imagine the stress involved in dealing with family members, friends, and coworkers who, although they may be sympathetic, call upon you to explain—over and over again—what the condition is all about or what the rationale is behind your new routines and restrictions.

YOUR FAMILY

If you have always enjoyed a communicative relationship with your spouse or significant other, openly sharing life's ups and downs and discussing both positive and negative feelings, this pattern is likely to continue as you go through the rigors of lymphedema treatment. Even couples who do not discuss emotional issues in this way may enjoy good relationships. They may intuitively understand each other, and each may empathize with the plight of the other, but verbal communication is not part of their style.

Often, however, when deeply troubling events occur, a lack of communication can lead to misunderstanding. If one partner is suffering but does not explain what is bothering him or her, the other partner may feel left out. If, on the other hand, the afflicted partner expresses all of his or her emotions, but does not receive the needed or expected response, he or she may feel abandoned. Now, more than ever, communication is paramount. While most people know this, at least on an intellectual level, it can be very difficult to change your essential nature or ingrained habits when it comes to dealing with others.

As you face the new challenges your condition imposes, there are some basic ground rules that can help you go a long way toward establishing the kind of atmosphere in which the needs of both partners and other family members are met. First, for the person with lymphedema:

• Remember that no one can help you if he or she is unaware of your needs. Don't expect people to be able to read your mind.

• If you need time to rest or temporary relief from some of your chores, express these needs in ways that your partner or family will understand. Try to avoid sounding angry or as if you are accusing the other person of something. For instance, you might say, "I'm not feeling well right now, and even making supper seems overwhelming to me. I'd appreciate as much help as you can give me." Or, "My arm feels swollen and heavy and I feel fatigued. I'm sorry I'll have to miss [the card game, the parent/teacher meeting, whatever], but

I'll be very interested in hearing from you what takes place." This kind of communication plainly tells the other person what the problem is, how it makes you feel, and the ways in which he or she can help you.

• Try to feel as benevolent toward yourself as you would like others to feel toward you. It is not uncommon for people who have enjoyed good health to feel angry at themselves when an illness makes them unable to be as vital as they once were. Now is the time for you to be as compassionate and patient with yourself as you have been with your children, your partner, and others you have helped in times of trouble.

For the family members of the person with lymphedema:

• Remember that illness—particularly if it involves discomfort, pain, and anxiety about treatment—can affect the personality of the person who suffers from the condition. Even someone who is ordinarily upbeat and resilient can feel so uncomfortable and demoralized that his or her optimism seems lost at this time.

• Try to learn as much as possible about your loved one's condition, not only for your own knowledge, but so that you can be a valuable resource. There are numerous stories of family members who were the first to find out about helpful treatments or who became important advocates for their loved ones because they had sought to become knowledgeable about the condition in question.

• Instead of waiting to be asked to help, volunteer to do the small things that let your loved one know you empathize with his or her discomfort. Prop up the pillows on the bed, make a cup of tea, buy a small gift (a book, flowers, a magazine)—whatever you know the person will appreciate.

• Ask your loved one how he or she feels. You may not be able to cure the physical condition, but your listening will be good medicine nevertheless.

Dealing with your children, and explaining to them that you have a serious problem that you must deal with every hour of every day, can be a particular challenge. For many children, a parent's illness is burdensome. In some instances, children are called upon to help out and even sacrifice their normal pleasures or curtail their usual schedules in the service of extra chores. In other cases, children are kept in the dark because their parents want to spare them worry. Either circumstance can cause resentment and guilt.

It is a good idea to discuss your concerns openly with your children. Even very young children sense when there is a problem in the family. It is better to bring that problem out in the open, before your children come up with an explanation that is worse than what is actually going on. Explain to your children, in terms they can understand, what is happening, what caused your lymphedema, and what you are doing about it. It is encouraging for children to learn that their parents are seekers of solutions. If you are upset or frustrated in finding good treatments or because of the discomfort of the condition, explain this as well. Dealing with the known—for both children and adults—is easier than dealing with the unknown. And definitely enlist the help of your children's teachers; they will thank you for helping them to help your children through this difficult time. You may also wish to consult one of the many books available to help parents reassure their children during times of trouble, such as Kathleen McCue's *How To Help Children Through A Parent's Serious Illness* (St. Martin's Press, 1996).

If, despite the best efforts of everyone concerned, relationships within the family are becoming increasingly strained and difficult, do not hesitate to seek additional help and support. Psychiatrists, psychologists, marriage and family therapists, and other mental health practitioners have helped many people to work through their problems and gain valuable insight, resulting in strengthened family bonds and a more positive outlook on life (the subject of professional help and psychological support will be discussed in detail in Chapter 9).

SEXUALITY

One of the most difficult problems that lymphedema poses involves sexuality. Because of the pain and discomfort of the condition, long-term sexual problems can arise if complete decongestive physiotherapy is not undertaken to relieve its symptoms. In addition, like any serious illness, lymphedema often consumes the energy and thoughts of those who suffer from it. It is not uncommon for people with lymphedema to feel a lack of sexual interest, even though they often feel a great need to be reassured by cuddling and touching. Then, too, there is the problem of feeling too self-conscious for physical intimacy because of a swollen arm or leg. Your partner may tell you, "You're still beautiful to me," but these words may not nullify your negative feelings about the way you think you appear.

If lymphedema affects your sexuality, intimacy can become strained and your husband, wife, or lover may seem distant or unaware of your needs. He or she may even become angry and resentful. Try to be open about your feelings, and ask that your partner be open about his or hers as well. Tell your partner what you expect in terms of sexual intimacy. This can go a long way toward lessening your self-consciousness and keeping your relationship strong. And always remember that there is a lot more to sexuality than a perfectly shaped arm or leg!

A good relationship is rarely adversely affected by lymphedema or by a temporary lack of sexual desire. Many couples, in fact, become closer during times of stress. If, however, changes in your sexual life become a source of difficulty and you feel you need help, there are numerous books available on the subjects of sexuality and the importance of touch, romance, and other forms of sexual communication. (See the Resources section at the end of the book for recommended reading on the subject.)

There are a number of other issues related to sexuality that can accompany lymphedema as well. If you have not had treatment, or if you have had treatment that worsened the condition, you may have developed genital lymphedema. This is a serious and devastating potential complication of primary and some secondary lymphedemas. Women who have had pelvic surgery usually have many pelvic lymph nodes removed, which may lead to swelling in the legs and genitalia. Men who have had lymph nodes removed and/or radiation for prostate or other types of cancer may experience genital swelling. Pelvic infections such as abscesses and recurrent limb infections may also result in genital lymphedema. Because it affects a part of the body that many people are uncomfortable talking about or seeking treatment for, its sufferers all too often try to ignore it and do not discuss it, even with their doctors or those closest to them. But the good news about this understandably demoralizing and uncomfortable condition is that it can usually be treated successfully with a combination of therapies, including the wearing of a compression garment. Treatment is most likely to be successful if undertaken as soon as symptoms begin.

When a flare-up of genital lymphedema occurs, the skin may become weepy and the area tender, sore, and swollen. Understandably, most people with this condition are simply not in the mood for sex.

Yet they may feel a greater than usual need for comfort and close-
ness. Of course, this is possible. Intimacy doesn't necessarily involve
sexual intercourse. Holding, touching, and snuggling are also ways
to be close and loving. Don't be shy about asking your partner for
this kind of loving comfort.

Often, certain warning signals occur before such flare-ups—a cut
in the skin, an area that feels warmer to the touch than surrounding
areas, or a sign of swelling. This should never be a watch-and-wait
situation. If you seek aggressive treatment with high doses of antibiotics, you may be able to avert a full-blown case of genital lymphedema. If it occurs in spite of your best efforts, conscientiously following the treatment regimen prescribed by your doctor or lymphedema therapist will eventually bring relief.

If you are not in a relationship, you will no doubt worry about
meeting someone and having to explain what lymphedema is, the
purpose of your compression garment, and why you have anxieties
about small things, such as a minor cut or going to the beach. As in
all new relationships, the best policy is to play it by ear, get to know
the person until you are comfortable with him or her, and then share
whatever you feel at ease sharing. Remember, you're the same person inside as you were before getting lymphedema.

Whatever type of sexual issues you encounter as a result of lymphedema, sexuality is a subject that can be spoken about openly in
psychotherapy or a support group, where everyone is in the same
boat and has the same misgivings. Actually, it is not uncommon for
the issue of sexuality, anxiety-provoking as it may be, to also have a
humorous side that can lighten both the general atmosphere and
your own mood. Support groups are particularly helpful when it
comes to discussing subjects that would be the most taboo anywhere
else, such as genital lymphedema. In meeting people who have the
same condition you do and who are willing to share the ways they
have coped with it, you will—probably for the first time—be among
those who understand the full implications of lymphedema and the
gravity of your feelings.

If you cannot find a support group or choose not to join one (or to
see a therapist), there is a lot you can do on your own to deal with
your darker feelings. Some are as simple as reading a funny book or
seeing comedic movies. Laughter stimulates the brain's endorphins,
which elevate mood and bring about feelings of well-being. Also,
talk, talk, talk. Talk to a trusted friend or coworker, to a hotline volunteer, or to a close neighbor. Talk is therapeutic, and often leads to

new coping behaviors and a new outlook. Even if the person you talk to is just "a pair of friendly ears," as one woman we know calls her support system, talk is still valuable. Sometimes, after all, what you really want is somebody simply to listen.

FRIENDS AND COWORKERS

When dealing with friends and coworkers, keep in mind that most people probably want to help, but they may not know where to begin. The policy of speaking openly, therefore, applies not only to your spouse, children, and other family members, but also to your friends and coworkers. If you are undergoing lymphedema treatment, or if you need assistance with some of your everyday activities, let those who offer to help know that they can car-pool your children, do some errands for you, fill in for you at work while you're away, or help out in other ways.

Lymphedema treatment is a time-consuming proposition, so you should discuss with your employer arrangements for sick time. Ask if you can borrow against current or future sick days, if necessary, during your lymphedema treatments. If something in the nature of your work may have to be modified to accommodate your new requirements, discuss this with your employer as well, and have your doctor write him or her a letter explaining what is required and why. Don't forget, it is illegal for you to be fired because of ill health! If you feel you are being harassed on the job because of your illness, contact your union representative or your state legislator about your rights.

Remember also that in 1990, the Americans With Disabilities Act became law, providing protection to the estimated 48 million Americans with disabilities. This law guarantees equal opportunity in employment and equal access to public services, transportation, and accommodations; services provided by private entities; and telecommunication services. It protects anyone who has a physical and/or mental impairment that substantially limits his or her functioning in a "major life activity" (including caring for oneself, walking, seeing, hearing, speaking, breathing, learning, and/or working), and requires that employers make "reasonable accommodations" in your tasks and/or environment to enable you to do your work. If you suffer from lymphedema to the extent that any of your major life activities is impaired, you may qualify for the protections this law offers. If speaking to your employer is not effective in bringing about needed accommodations, you may need the services of an attorney to speak for you.

It can be emotionally taxing to have to adopt a whole new way of dealing with people and circumstances that once posed only "normal" problems. Most people with lymphedema, however, are adults who already have a good track record in making their feelings and needs known. If you have held a job, been in a relationship, raised children, or simply negotiated the ups and downs of life, you are equipped to meet this challenge as well. It may take some new phrasing and rethinking, and there may be a few bumps in the road, but you can do it!

9

Your Emotions

The new rules you must learn when you have lymphedema—actually a new way of living—are often made more difficult by emotional feelings ranging from anger to sadness to fear. Even having an essentially optimistic nature or a positive attitude does not preclude feelings of depression or anxiety. These are normal reactions to abnormal circumstances, part and parcel of the human condition.

Today, because of the hectic nature of modern life, the unrelenting expectations of family and career, and the equally rigorous demands of treatment, many people with lymphedema find themselves literally too busy to get depressed for long periods of time. Even so, they may find themselves weighed down by feelings of despair from time to time.

It is important to be concerned about your emotions as well as your physical problems when you have a chronic condition such as lymphedema, because your mental state has a very real influence on your body, particularly on your immune system. A great deal of research exists showing that people who undergo psychotherapy after traumatic events, and who have the opportunity to talk openly and express their emotions, fare better not only emotionally, but physically.[1] In a 1986 University of Pennsylvania Cancer Center study involving 359 patients with advanced cancer, it was found that those with positive, combative attitudes toward their conditions lived longer than those patients who gave up.[2]

Other studies have found that feelings of helplessness (which are often found in people who are depressed) may hinder the ability of the immune system to function normally, whereas feeling in control of a stressful situation keeps the immune system functioning as it should. Recent studies by both psychologists and immunologists have revealed that a person who is taught to look at life more optimistically can boost his or her immune response.[3]

It is therefore vital to look at your emotions as part of your condition, and to recognize and deal appropriately with your feelings.

DEPRESSION

Depression is common after the onset of lymphedema, as is the anxiety that can seem to pervade every minute of every day—panic every time you get a minor cut or burn, and fear of infection and increased swelling. It is no wonder so many lymphedema sufferers find themselves withdrawing, abandoning daily workouts or diet regimens, avoiding people and activities they once enjoyed, or discontinuing—by necessity—even pleasurable pursuits, such as exercise classes or recreational sports. Sometimes the symptoms of lymphedema are so debilitating, people are forced to leave their employment as well. If you developed the condition as a result of surgery for cancer or some other serious health problem, lymphedema serves as a constant reminder of the trauma you experienced. The discomfort lymphedema causes, the physical limitations it imposes, the altered appearance it brings about, and all the adjustments it requires—all of these can undermine the spirits of even the most optimistic person.

There is a difference between reactive depression—a transient feeling of sadness that results from a particular event in your life—and clinical depression, which often signals that a change in your body's chemistry has taken place. Stress and sadness assault the system. They are intruders that often interrupt the normal ebb and flow of life. Yet it is common to misinterpret depression, to blame the fact that you are feeling down on the weather or a broken appliance or an irritating conversation.

A good way to assess if, indeed, you are suffering from depression is to ask yourself if you have been experiencing any of the following:

- Chronic feelings of sadness or despair.

- Loss of appetite (or overeating).

- Oversleeping.

- Withdrawal from friends, family members, and coworkers.

- Atypical irritability or anger.

- An inability to concentrate.

- Little or no interest in sex.

- Lack of normal energy.

- Uncontrollable crying.

- Brooding about the past.

- Feelings of hopelessness.

- Mood swings.

- Deteriorating personal relationships.

- Thoughts of suicide.

If you have been experiencing four or more of these symptoms, chances are you are suffering from depression. Sometimes, though, depression may be masked. This means that you may act unusually upbeat and make yourself busy every minute of the day in order to cover up your feelings of sadness.

The good news about depression is that it is a treatable condition. Through short- or long-term psychotherapy or medication, or a combination of both, you can break free of the oppressive feelings that are dragging you down and making sunny skies seem gray. There are even herbal remedies that may help. In Germany, the herb St. John's wort is more commonly prescribed for depression than Prozac! Whatever approach you prefer, we recommend consulting your doctor or a mental health expert for assistance. To find a mental health practitioner, ask your doctor or lymphedema therapist for a referral, call your local medical society, or simply ask a friend who may have had a similar experience.

ANGER

One of the most difficult emotions for many people to acknowledge is anger, and people with lymphedema experience plenty of anger— anger at the intractable nature of the condition, at the ways in which it affects their lives, at the inconveniences it imposes every day, at the difficulty in finding treatment, and at the arduousness of treatment itself. It is frequently impossible for those suffering from lymphedema to express this rage to family and friends. If they do, it is often misunderstood, or places loved ones in the awkward (and helpless) position of not being able to do anything to make the situation better, a position from which they may retreat. This can lead to feelings of abandonment on the part of the person with lymphedema, and with that, more depression and anger.

Once expressed, however, anger can actually make you feel good! It is not uncommon for people to say that once they were able to get angry, they not only felt better, but they were able to channel their anger in productive ways, either personally or politically. It is important, though, to find ways and settings in which you can express your anger constructively, not destructively. In support groups or psychotherapy, be they short- or long-term, you can let your tears flow and your rage find expression.

FEAR

Dread, horror, panic. These are some of the feelings that people with lymphedema face when confronted not only with their frightening symptoms but with the knowledge that this condition will be with them for the rest of their lives.

If you have ever had these feelings, you have plenty of company. No one with lymphedema really escapes the fear factor. In fact, fear is a perfectly appropriate emotion since so little is known about this condition and the effective treatments that do exist are not offered to many lymphedema patients.

It is *not knowing* that causes fear. Think about the people you know who have been diagnosed with diabetes or seizure disorders or even cancer. "This is what we know about the condition," the doctor says, "and this is how we can treat it or fight it." While the doctor may not offer any guarantees, he or she says the magic words: "This is how we can treat it or fight it." For people with these conditions, there are at least *some* answers. For people with lymphedema, however, there often seem to be *no* answers.

By knowing that there *are* answers, you can conquer fear. True, there is no cure—no magic wand you can wave to make lymphedema go away. But as you now know, there are many effective strategies you can use to diminish swelling, reduce pain, minimize infection, protect yourself in everyday life, and turn fear and depression into hope and optimism.

SELF-BLAME

In their book *Getting Well Again* (J.P. Tarcher, 1978), O. Carl Simonton and Stephanie Simonton address "the idea of personal responsibility" in the onset or progression of disease.[4] They make a clear distinction between the concepts of responsibility and blame. Responsibility, they say, is a starting point for recognizing the potential for change, whereas blame induces unnecessary (and unproductive) guilt and other negative feelings.

While taking charge and empowering yourself with information can be positive steps in getting well, to many people, the flip side of the "I-can-do-something-about-my-illness" attitude is the idea that they must somehow have brought the disease or condition upon themselves—a feeling many lymphedema patients erroneously hold. In the view of Dr. Bernie Siegel, bestselling author of books on self-healing, there should be no self-blame, only the opportunity to utilize your resources in adapting new strategies, including unorthodox remedies.[5] In other words, it's a waste of your time and energy to ruminate about what caused your lymphedema. Whether it was an accident of birth, a traumatic injury, or disease—if you inherited a defective gene, had the misfortune to get cancer, even if you were drunk when you got involved in an automobile accident that injured your lymphatic system—none of that matters. What matters is what you do about your condition now. This includes using many of the strategies and resources you have used before to solve problems and exploring every credible and available treatment possible to manage your condition.

SELF-CONSCIOUSNESS

Because a lymphedematous limb that has swelled to three, four, or even five times its normal size, is not "pretty," there is always a degree of self-consciousness, if not downright embarrassment, that comes along with this condition. It is upsetting to see your limb in this condition. Like a teenager with an unsightly blemish on his or her face, the person with lymphedema often thinks that the whole world is looking only at his or her arm or leg. It is not uncommon for people with lymphedema to become so despairing that they mentally dissociate their lymphedematous limbs from the rest of their bodies, pretending that they doesn't exist. One woman we know went so far as to purchase a sponge on a long handle so that when she took a shower, she didn't have to touch her arm.

While searching for solutions, patients are faced with the reality of lymphedema each time they wake up in the morning and do something as unremarkable as selecting an outfit to wear. To women who have had a breast removed, the trauma of seeing a lymphedematous arm is sometimes more upsetting than a missing breast. The loss of a breast can be dealt with by wearing a prosthesis or having reconstructive surgery. But a ballooning arm cannot be concealed. There is no hiding an advanced case of lymphedema, and no way to wear the lingerie, bathing suits, or blouses that now sit in their bureaus or hang in their closets. We have met numerous people with lymphedema who said they wept as they gave away wardrobes that no longer fit or abandoned activities in which they could no longer participate.

For many people with lymphedema, recapturing the feelings of attractiveness and sexiness that were once taken for granted is extremely difficult. They certainly don't consider this new reality the mere inconvenience they have been told to consider it. One of the most demoralizing thing about lymphedema is the toll it takes on your self-esteem. When an arm or leg swells to several times its normal size, the clothes you once chose with care may no longer fit, or they may be constricting. There are so many fashion choices out there today that finding new, appropriate clothing that is also fashionable should not be a problem. What may be a problem is adjusting to clothes that you believe are not "you."

Now is the time to subscribe to Look Good—Feel Better. This is a program developed jointly by the American Cancer Society and the cosmetics industry to teach postsurgical and posttrauma patients to utilize clothing and makeup in creative ways. By using cosmetic enhancements, clothes, and accessories such as scarves, you can alter or camouflage the appearance of a perceived defect. While this program does not specifically address the disfigurement of lymphedema, it does lift the spirits. Become determined to find suitable cover-up clothing in colors and styles that suit your taste, even if the result is a wardrobe quite different from the one you have been used to. Outside trappings will not magically eliminate inside pain, but knowing that you look your best will help to boost your mood and self-confidence.

PSYCHOTHERAPY AND SUPPORT GROUPS

Oppressive emotional feelings can leave you feeling lonely and isolated. It is wonderful, but not all that common, to be able to express all your emotions to your family and friends. But many people believe they are burdening others by speaking about their problems, and sometimes even those closest to you don't know exactly how to respond. In addition, many people find it difficult to express their emotions in words—to express feelings that may have been unfamiliar to them for most of their lives. In the past, you may have been able to cheer yourself up with a pep talk or by taking some positive action. Similarly, friends and family members may have been able to rouse you out of a state of sadness by being extra loving or by saying the right thing. Now, however, you may find yourself unresponsive to such efforts. If this happens, friends and family members often feel at a loss and give up trying.

Dealing with your feelings in the atmosphere of understanding and support afforded by a professional therapist or support group can help you face the stages of emotional pain—fear, denial, anxiety, and grieving—that go along with any loss, and also to deal more effectively with your spouse and children, other family members, and friends. Here is where you can discuss your hidden fears about the future; your anger and depression about what has happened to you; anxieties about your appearance and feeling sexually undesirable; the pain of having to deal with stares or insensitive remarks; and all of your other feelings—feelings you may be withholding from family members, friends, even doctors. In these settings, you can revisit important issues again and again, without the fear of taxing those around you. In fact, in group settings, the person who expresses an emotion often finds that it taps the deepest feelings of other group members and allows them to vent their own feelings for the first time.

Another benefit of a weekly session with a psychotherapist or participation in a support group is that it gets you out, away from your usual surroundings. Often, especially at the beginning, this can be the highlight of your week and can leave you feeling energized and optimistic about the future. A further benefit is the potential for joining forces with other support group members to become politically active, if that is your bent (this will be discussed further in Chapter 11). Because lymphedema is still not well known, and demands new research, funding for research, and greater public awareness, it is probable that you will find members who are ready, willing, and able to write letters, lobby legislators, attend rallies and meetings, and get the word out about lymphedema. Many people have forged lifelong friendships in such groups and, working together, have made a difference in their own lives and in society at large.

If you want to try working with a psychological counselor, how do you find one and what can you expect from consulting such a person? Extremely lucky people never ask these questions. They talk to their mothers, fathers, grandparents, aunts, uncles, or siblings, and they receive all the support and advice they need. But for most of us, these traditional sources of support are not there. We don't want to burden our parents (or they were never "there for us" to begin with), our grandparents wouldn't get it at all, we've lost touch with our aunts and uncles, and our siblings are busy with their own lives. In large part, this is the modern age! And in today's world, people often turn to professionals for support and advice. There are different types of professionals in the mental health field that may be of help, among them psychiatrists, psychologists, clinical social workers, psychiatric nurse specialists, and individual or family counselors.

Psychiatrists are medical doctors who have taken four years of extra study in the specialty after medical school. Many study even longer to become proficient at psychoanalysis, a technique that seeks to uncover the *why* of a person's feelings and behavior and explain them in terms of early childhood experiences. Once you realize why you have certain emotional and behavioral habits, the theory goes, you can be liberated from them if you choose to be. Traditional psychoanalysis typically involves four or five sessions a week in which you explore your unconscious; you speak about your life and feelings in a free-floating way, and the psychiatrist listens. Sessions cost between $100 and $250 an hour. With today's managed-care approach to health coverage, psychoanalysis is mostly for people who have lots of money.

Psychologists usually major in psychology in undergraduate school and then go on to get master's and doctoral degrees in clinical psychology—that is, the treatment of patients. Some clinical psychologists specialize in psychoanalytic therapy. Others utilize cognitive and behavioral therapy, an approach in which the patient learns to substitute new, healthier thought and behavior patterns for older, unhealthy ones. Still others take an eclectic approach that includes elements of many different psychological schools of thought. Psychologists' fees range from $75 to $150 per hour.

Clinical social workers also treat people with emotional problems. A clinical social worker usually has a bachelor's degree in one of the social sciences plus a three-year clinical master's degree. Like psychologists, clinical social workers can use a variety of therapeutic approaches. Their fees range from $75 to $100 per hour. Psychiatric nurse specialists have four-year nursing degrees, with an emphasis on the ways in which physiological and psychological conditions are related, and masters' or doctoral degrees in mental health practice. Their fees range from $75 to $100 per hour. There are also practitioners who have obtained one- or two-year degrees in individual or family counseling; their fees range from $50 to $75 per hour. And many clergy members have either taken courses in counseling or learned counseling techniques through experience. A clergy counselor may or may not charge a fee, or may ask for a voluntary donation to the house of worship in exchange for his or her services.

No matter what type of practitioner you decide to work with, you should feel that your therapist understands you, empathizes with your plight, and is able to help you tap your own resources to make good choices for yourself. Will that person solve your problems? No. Will he or she help you to sort out your feelings? Yes, if you are receptive to this type of treatment—although be warned, it can be difficult work! But if you feel a therapist doesn't fit your bill, look further. Even the "best" or most highly recommended therapist may not be right for *you*. Trust your feelings. If you feel like seeking help elsewhere, do so, and be confident that you have made the right choice. The right fit for you may be just around the corner.

Support groups come in all varieties. The more structured groups are usually led by professionals, such as social workers or psychiatric nurses, who have special training in group dynamics. In these groups, specific topics are scheduled for discussion and the leader guides the interaction. Other groups are more free-wheeling, and members spontaneously decide on the topic or topics to be discussed.

Some groups continue to meet for months or years; in other cases, members decide on a limited time span, usually six to twelve weeks. Whatever the nature of the group, there are no hard and fast rules about how you must participate. Some people find they benefit most from sitting and listening, others from speaking out. The one unwritten, but highly honored, ethic of any support group is respect for other members' confidentiality.

There are no foolproof guidelines for choosing a support group. The most important element is that you feel welcome and comfortable. Even though you may feel particularly vulnerable at this time, trust your own judgment. If for any reason the group you initially selected doesn't feel right, try another. Don't abandon this potentially helpful path because of one bad experience.

In many instances, people who see psychotherapists or who join support groups bring back to their families the insights they have gained, as well as helpful strategies that improve family relationships. In addition, there are many psychotherapists and support groups that encourage the presence of family members, or that have separate meetings for spouses or teenagers. If you would like to join a support group but cannot locate one in your area, consider starting one. (*See* Starting a Lymphedema Support Group, page 153.)

Though support groups and psychotherapy can both be valuable for helping you deal with your emotions, they do not fill exactly the same need. Specifically, a support group should not be seen as a substitute for psychotherapy. Support groups are excellent for helping people to cope with chronic illness and its effects. Deeper or longer term problems, such as relationship problems or serious mental illness, may require psychotherapeutic treatment.

It can be overwhelming to consider the many ways that lymphedema will change your life. Yet the changes in attitude and behavior it demands of you are things you have probably experienced, in one way or another, at other times in your life. Remember leaving home? Getting married? Starting a new job? Having a baby? As most people know, all of these seemingly ordinary events are not ordinary at all. All of them involve great personal changes and adjustments. And you did them!

Taking things one step at a time, one day at a time, is the trick. Will you forget a regimen or a warning or a new way of thinking now and then? Will you need help and support along the way? Will you sometimes feel sad or fed up? Yes, yes, and yes again—because that's human. We are not machines, and life is rarely without its ups and downs.

The most important thing to keep in mind is that help is available and that *you* can find that help. By taking control, asking the right questions, letting your doctors and therapists know that you wish to collaborate in your own treatment, making your lymphedema journey a one-step-at-a-time process, and seeking out an empathetic support system, you will learn to manage your condition successfully.

Starting a Lymphedema Support Group

If you cannot locate a lymphedema support group in your community, start one yourself! It might begin with only you and one other person, but it will be worth it.

Here are some guidelines for starting your own group:

• *Ask your doctor or lymphedema therapist to give your name and phone number to other patients who have or may be at risk for lymphedema. You might begin your relationships over the phone, sharing "war stories" and discussing ways to meet on a regular basis.*

• *Contact cancer support groups in your community and ask them to tell their members that you are starting a lymphedema support group and want to hear from them. Be sure to leave the telephone number where you can be reached, either at home or work.*

• *Get in touch with the nursing department of your local hospital and ask for nursing support for lymphedema and for the group you're starting. Registered nurses have been among the most ardent supporters of lymphedema patients, often initiating the pink-wristband policy in their hospitals and educating both patients and doctors about this condition.*

• *Place flyers in hospitals, doctors' offices, treatment centers, supermarkets, laundromats, and libraries, inviting people with lymphedema to contact you.*

• *Place an advertisement in your local newspaper or* Pennysaver *or other shopper's weekly. Many publications have free space for volunteer organizations. Also, contact your local radio station; many give free spots to advertise volunteer groups.*

• *If you cannot or do not want to hold meetings in your home, ask your local hospital, public library, or community center if they will donate a room once a month. Sometimes local restaurants are willing to do this. Houses of worship may also provide space either free or for a nominal fee.*

• *Open the group to all people who are suffering from or are at risk for lymphedema. If the group becomes too large, you may want to form specialized groups. You might form groups for women who have had breast cancer, for men, for people with primary lymphedema (adults and/or teens), or anything else there is a demand for, as well as for family members.*

• *If you have motivated volunteers and adequate financing, start a newsletter. This is always a help to those unable to attend regular meetings because of physical or emotional limitations. A pen-pal section is helpful for communication among members.*

• *Invite professional speakers to make presentations and answer your questions. Doctors, oncology nurses, social workers, lymphedema therapists, even compression-garment manufacturers have valuable expertise in lymphedema.*

Starting a support group does not require an immense amount of work. All it takes is the initiative of one person and the belief that the good that will come out of sharing experiences, resources, and feelings has value. A support group offers seemingly endless sources of helpful hints and seasoned advice, an opportunity to vent your feelings, and an introduction to people with whom you may form deep and lasting friendships and even, if you are so inclined, political-action alliances.

People who establish or join support groups invariably say the groups have given them the best ideas, advice, support, and encouragement. If you need additional help, don't hesitate to call the American Self-Help Clearinghouse (see the Resources section at the end of the book). This is an organization that provides information about finding an existing group or setting up your own. If you're hesitating, don't! You deserve it!

10

Insurance Issues

Every other day, it seems, another article appears in the press detailing the plight of a person who needs a bone-marrow transplant or some other complicated and potentially life-saving procedure, but cannot get it because his or her insurance company refuses to pay for it. Sometimes this is because the procedure is considered experimental or unproven, even if it is used routinely for people with other conditions. A similar fate befalls many people with lymphedema.

WHAT'S COVERED, WHAT'S NOT

High on the list of procedures most insurance companies don't cover is lymphedema therapy. Apparently, lymphedema—a widespread condition that requires lifelong treatment—is not considered important enough for insurance coverage.

Both in the United States and abroad, doctors and therapists treating lymphedema patients have written extensively on the effectiveness of manual lymph drainage (MLD) and complete decongestive physiotherapy (CDP). But for reasons known only to the medical and research establishments, few studies and clinical trials of these treatments have been conducted in the United States. This is problematic for lymphedema patients because it enables insurance companies to refuse to pay for the treatment on the basis that there is "no proof" of its effectiveness.

The result is that most people who suffer from lymphedema must pay out of pocket for treatments whose cost can approach a thousand dollars a day. Since few people can afford these extraordinarily expensive fees, many go without treatment and suffer needlessly while their symptoms worsen.

If all hospitals throughout the country had lymphedema clinics or treatment centers, these costs could be reduced dramatically. But that will not happen until lymphedema patients begin to bring the human and economic costs of this malady to public attention—or at least to the attention of their doctors, hospitals, insurance companies, and legislators.

Here is a scenario that may be familiar to you. After what seems like a million questions, phone calls, letters, and conversations, not to mention arduous investigation, you learn that treatment is, in fact, available, and you have found a treatment center and a person licensed and trained in lymphedema therapy. What a relief!

So far, all seems promising. Unfortunately, however, even these discoveries will not ensure that you get the treatment you need. Key to getting proper treatment by a qualified practitioner is your ability to afford it. In general, in order to qualify for insurance reimbursement, you must be treated by a licensed medical doctor, registered nurse, or physical or occupational therapist. A massage therapist trained and licensed in lymphedema therapy is not considered a "health professional" by insurance companies. Such practitioners are not even listed in the industry's ICD-9 codes, a classification system for diseases and procedures used by doctors and insurance companies. Even worse, the Current Procedural Terminology (CPT) code, a system developed by the American Medical Association (AMA) for the purpose of identifying clinical conditions and assisting the insurance industry in covering those conditions, doesn't even list lymphedema as a condition. In effect, by not including it, the AMA is saying lymphedema doesn't exist! Needless to say, this is both shocking and dismaying to the millions of people who suffer from it. As one woman we know remarked, "If I take antibiotics for an infected pimple that goes away in three days, I'm covered by my medical insurance. My lymphedema never goes away and requires treatment after treatment, yet my insurance company acts as if they never heard of it!"

Then there are the necessary compression garments. Their cost is significant, and the garments last for only about six months before they need to be replaced. Some insurance companies will tell you that they cover the cost of compression sleeves and stockings, and some will, in fact, pay, but most do not. To say that this is unfair is an understatement. Lymphedema is a serious medical condition, and the compression sleeve or stocking that must be worn daily to relieve or diminish swelling and pain is the single most important item patients need. A limb that has been treated and reduced in size but left without the follow-up benefits of a compression garment will quickly fill up with fluid again.

THE INSURANCE NIGHTMARE

Increasing numbers of lymphedema patients are learning of and seeking MLD and CDP treatments and finding them effective. But encouraged as you may be to have finally found some relief, this is often the beginning of your own personal insurance nightmare. The ordeal usually begins after you find a center or person licensed and trained to administer lymphedema treatment, and either you or your doctor requests authorization from your insurance carrier.

Many times, insurance companies will tell you they are presenting a request to their medical review team. Months go by, and the insurance company continues to ask for additional information—well after they have received all the information available and relevant to the case. In the meantime, the condition becomes worse. Many people, at this point desperate for help, find someone trained in the treatment, usually a massage therapist who qualifies neither for state licensing nor for medical insurance coverage. Generally, these therapists charge less for treatment than lymphedema centers do, but their fees are not reimbursable by insurance carriers. This places you in a no-win situation; you can either avail yourself of desperately needed treatment that is not reimbursable, or you can forgo treatment altogether because of the prohibitive cost.

Sally's story is typical. She underwent surgery for breast cancer, and midway through her postsurgery radiation treatments, her arm began to swell. When she leaned against the edge of a table or on an armrest, she was horrified to notice an indentation, really a deep gully, on the underside of her forearm. She had never been told this might happen, and was reassured by her doctor that it would go away. "Just raise your arm," he advised her.

After conducting her own research, Sally found a lymphedema center located an hour from her home. She asked her primary-care physician to write a letter of medical necessity to her insurance carrier, so that the cost of her treatments would be reimbursed. She waited and waited to hear from her insurer, to no avail. Finally, she called and was told that they needed more information.

This scenario went on for months, as Sally supplied the insurance company with volumes of information only to be asked for more. Then there was no more; she had sent the company absolutely everything that related to her case. Finally, she understood—the insurance company was stalling!

By this time, Sally's arm was so swollen and painful, she decided to be fitted for a sleeve, after which she sought the services of a massage therapist who had the credentials to administer manual lymph drainage. All along, Sally feared that if she continued to wait for her insurance company to authorize treatments, her arm would swell beyond repair. The director of the treatment center she wanted to go to told her that, two years before, he had contacted dozens of insurance companies (including the one providing Sally's coverage), and they had claimed they didn't have a "patient load" for the specialized type of lymphedema treatment the center offered. In other words, they claimed there was not enough consumer demand to justify covering the treatment. In light of the high incidence of breast cancer and the increasing incidence of lymphedema in recent years, Sally found this incomprehensible. And she knew it wasn't true. Not only was her insurance company aware of her case, but the nurses in its health-services department had called her numerous times for advice about other plan members with lymphedema.

On one occasion, the insurance company told her their plan allowed for her to receive lymphedema treatment from a physical therapist on their list of approved practitioners. But by this time Sally had made herself extremely knowledgeable about lymphedema treatment and, after checking the therapist's credentials and experience, learned that she had none in lymphedema treatment.

The only treatment the company agreed to reimburse Sally for was the pump. It is relevant to mention here that insurance companies in the United States consider the pump the norm in the treatment of lymphedema, despite the fact that it has inherent dangers and that other treatments have proven highly effective.

Ultimately, Sally paid twelve hundred dollars for treatment at the lymphedema center that should have been—but wasn't—available through her medical insurance plan. To this day, she is fighting with her insurance company for fair and timely reimbursement.

DEALING WITH YOUR INSURANCE COMPANY

It is demoralizing and infuriating to pay regular premiums to a health-insurance company only to learn that when you need treatment, the company doesn't cover it. Unfortunately, it is all too often the case. Here are some ways to redress this outrage:

• Call your insurance carrier (on their toll-free number, if they have one) and ask if lymphedema treatment is covered or is excluded from the policy. Some carriers omit the names of participating lymphedema specialists in their provider listings, making it difficult to find out that they cover the treatment. We know of several treatment centers that have been participating in major insurance company plans for some time yet are still not listed in those companies' literature.

• In petitioning for coverage of lymphedema treatment, provide your insurance company with well-documented information supporting the effectiveness of lymphedema therapy from articles in medical journals, with corroborating data from your doctor, as well as with a description of your own experiences with the condition.

• If lymphedema treatment is covered by your insurer, ask what portion of the payment you will be responsible for (the copayment), as well as the maximum the company will allow for ongoing treatment. Also, ask if the coverage provides for outpatient or inpatient treatment.

• Every time you speak with an insurance company representative, write down his or her name, the date and time of your call, and the information you receive. If you get a verbal agreement for coverage, request that the representative send it to you in writing. If you don't receive it, follow up with additional requests until you get what you need.

• Check with your doctor about his or her experience with insurance coverage for lymphedema treatment and how other patients have dealt with their claims. He or she may be aware of strategies that have worked for other patients seeking reimbursement for lymphedema treatment, or of other insurance companies that will cover this service.

• If your insurance company denies you reimbursement for a compression garment, have your physician write a letter of medical necessity explaining the importance of the garment to effective treatment. This should be accompanied by a letter of your own, explaining what happens to your limb if you do not wear the sleeve or stocking. In some cases, these letters are all that is needed to get reimbursement.

• Pumps are generally covered under most insurance plans. But, as we have seen, great care must be taken in obtaining proper instructions before using a pump. Being reimbursed for this treatment will not compensate for the problems that may ensue if the pump is used incorrectly. Continue to press for coverage of complete decongestive physiotherapy. If your insurance company does not cover the cost even of the pump, ask your doctor to write a letter of medical necessity explaining why you need this treatment and include a letter of your own, explaining the value of the pump in treating your lymphedema.

• If treatment is denied after you have tried all these strategies, keep fighting. Inform your insurance company that you are prepared to fight for coverage of lymphedema treatment, and that you will contact your elected state representatives, your state's insurance committee, and an attorney, if necessary. Then do so!

• If you should leave your job *for any reason*, be sure to continue your insurance coverage under the Consolidated Omnibus Budget Reconciliation Act, or COBRA. This provision gives you the right to participate in your former employer's group insurance on your own for up to eighteen months after you leave your job. COBRA coverage may be expensive, but if you are unable to work or have difficulty finding another job, it is definitely worth it.

It is unlikely that your insurance company will deny coverage for a second or third opinion. But they may deny coverage for "off-label" use of drugs (the practice of prescribing a drug approved by the FDA for one condition to treat a different condition), for "experimental" treatments (which many consider lymphedema therapy to be), or for "preexisting conditions" (which can be a problem if you must change insurance carriers). In such cases you may need the services of an attorney who specializes in patient advocacy or insurance problems. If you do not currently have an attorney, or do not know where to find the kind of lawyer who specializes in patient advocacy or insurance problems, call your local Bar Association or a nearby law school, or look under "Lawyer Referral Service" in the Yellow Pages of your local telephone directory.

You and your lawyer may first try a couple of simple strategies to solve these problems. You might write to your insurance company, explaining that you intend to contact a lawyer. Or you might have your lawyer send the company a letter stating that he or she intends to press a claim on your behalf. Sometimes, this is all that's needed.

But be prepared to be persistent in pressing your claim. An insurance company may try to wait you out, stalling until you give up and stop fighting. If they know you are serious and unlikely to give up, they are more likely to change their tune.

In addition to pursuing the company directly, don't hesitate to call your local newspaper or a local television or radio reporter and go public with your insurance problem. Some of the most dramatic insurance-company policy reversals in the last decade have occurred when patients have brought their plights to public attention.

THE ROLE OF THE LYMPHEDEMA THERAPIST

One of the problems that keeps people from getting reimbursed for lymphedema treatment and management is that there are no recognized codes for manual lymph drainage (MLD) or complete decongestive physiotherapy (CDP) among the insurance industry (see page 156). Because of this, the widespread and chronic condition of lymphedema itself is rarely recognized in the medical-insurance world.

Rarely, but *not never.* There are determined and inventive professionals in lymphedema treatment who have succeeded in devising ways of offering their patients the best in lymphedema therapy—which includes not only MLD but bandages and compression garments—*and* ensuring that the therapy is reimbursed. To be sure, this process can be frustrating, to therapists as well as to patients, but until insurance coverage for lymphedema therapy becomes the rule, a diligent, determined therapist or lymphedema center staff member who is prepared to act as an advocate may be your best ally in obtaining payment for necessary treatment.

One example of this type of advocacy is provided by The Lymphedema Connection of Pittsburgh, Pennsylvania (also known by the apt acronym TLC), which succeeded in coming to an agreement for coverage with a major health-maintenance organization (HMO). First, TLC scrutinized the insurance industry's CPT codes to find appropriate pathways for reimbursement. Then they dispatched several members of their staff to make the case for covering the proper management of lymphedema—including coverage for bandages, compression garments, and other necessary products—before the HMO's executive directors. To ensure their credibility, they sent staff members with unquestionable credentials, among them a plastic surgeon, a physical therapist, and a registered nurse (the latter two also were certified manual lymphatic therapists).

In several meetings, the TLC representatives stressed what is involved in providing the best care for people with lymphedema, and pointed out how a true lymphedema center's services were very different from the treatments offered by other practitioners and suppliers. Just a few months after beginning this informational campaign, TLC finalized an agreement with the HMO that allowed for coverage not only of manual lymph drainage, but for the products that go along with it.

Other lymphedema therapists have explored other options in advocating for their patients. In 1997, administrators of the lymphedema therapy program at the University of New York Medical Hospital and Medical Center at Stony Brook applied to a number of philanthropic foundations for grants to pay for medical services for their patients. In their proposals, they spelled out the degree to which comprehensive lymphedema treatment is often not covered by insurance companies and the fact that this places on patients the burden of paying for any uncovered portion of the treatment. To their (and their patients') delight, one foundation responded with a grant of $50,000. While the grant was for only one year, the facility may be able to have it extended. And at least for that year, patients at the facility were spared one of the many griefs that most lymphedema patients endure—and will continue to endure until insurance companies enact significant changes in their policies regarding coverage for treatment of this chronic condition.

If you have or are at risk for lymphedema, it may be a good idea to look for health insurance based on different companies' lymphedema coverage. If you find a lymphedema center and it seems that help is finally on the way, ask first which insurance plans it participates in, then investigate the possibility of switching coverage, if necessary. Conversely, it is wise to consider the attitude of practitioners toward assisting their patients with insurance issues. If you find a lymphedema therapist or facility that is a true advocate, willing to educate insurance companies about the need to cover lymphedema treatment, you are much more likely to be able to get the treatment you need.

GETTING THE TREATMENT YOU NEED

While you are petitioning your insurance company, you need treatment! If you don't have the ability to pay for it on your own, don't give up. There are other avenues that may be worth investigating.

Here are some suggestions:

• If your income is above the level that would qualify you for government assistance but you don't have the ability to pay for lymphedema therapy on your own, contact your local medical society and state legislators and tell them of your problem and your uninsured status. They may be able to help or offer useful referrals. Also, your doctor may be able to make special arrangements, such as allowing you to pay in small amounts over a long period of time rather than all at once.

• If you are seeking lymphedema treatment in a hospital, remember to take along a list of all your debts, including those for your mortgage, car payments, credit cards, and tuition bills. That way, if they question your financial status, you will be able to document your situation.

• Contact local fraternal organizations, social-service agencies, and church and synagogue groups that may offer financial help or know of other sources of such assistance.

• Contact local and national breast-cancer coalitions and agencies. Ask them to write letters to elected officials and insurance companies. It is always a good idea to provide these agencies with a sample letter to be sure that the issues you care about are included.

When illness strikes, it often seems that the very act of getting out of bed in the morning is a heroic accomplishment. When that is followed by arduous treatments, keeping up with the demands of one's career, and juggling domestic responsibilities, not to mention coping with the toll that exhaustion, anxiety, and depression take, it can seem like just too much to have to deal with an insurance company on top of it all. Even under the best of circumstances, this can be unpleasant—the hours of filling out forms, the back-and-forth phone calls, and then waiting to be reimbursed.

With lymphedema, however, this cannot be avoided. In fact, it is urgent! The sooner you find out whether or not your insurance company covers the cost of treatment, the sooner you can either begin treatment or begin fighting the system. Every effort you make to secure coverage for your lymphedema treatment will make a difference for you, and for other lymphedema patients who are waging the same battle.

11

Making a Difference

Most people who have lymphedema, or who are at risk of developing it, have already undergone the rigors of cancer surgery or a traumatic accident. During such sieges, it is not unusual to become philosophical, to think about the meaning of life, and to contemplate your own mortality.

Initially—and naturally—people focus on themselves: "What will happen to me?" "What will my treatments be like?" "Where can I find help?" But with the availability of treatments that can prolong life, many people return to health and vigor after serious illness, and more and more of them are turning outward, sharing their experiences with others and getting involved in a variety of activities to make a difference, not only to their own sense of well-being but to the larger society as well.

People with lymphedema know only too well how many things in "the system" need to be changed if their grievances are to be redressed and the experiences they have had are not to be encountered by others.

WHAT YOU CAN DO

It is common to think that one person cannot really make a difference. "But what can I do?" is usually the first question that springs to mind. In fact, there are many examples of how one person's efforts can bring about tremendous progress. In the arena of lymphedema, one of the most dramatic is that of Saskia R.J. Thiadens. In the 1980s, Saskia, a registered nurse, was operating a postoperative care facility. She found herself increasingly mystified by the swollen arms and legs of many of her patients, and frustrated that the limbs seemed so resistant to treatment. She embarked on her own research, which included several trips to Europe, and learned that this curiously resistant condition was called lymphedema. She also learned that there was more help available for lymphedema than her patients had been led to believe, and she became a certified lymphedema therapist.

Sacrificing a steady income, Saskia closed her facility and founded the National Lymphedema Network (NLN). Her goals: to provide education and guidance to lymphedema patients, health-care professionals, and the general public by disseminating information on the prevention and management of primary and secondary lymphedema; to standardize quality treatment for lymphedema patients nationwide; and to support research into the causes and possible alternative treatments for this long-neglected condition. Today, the NLN has some 3,800 patient, therapist, and professional dues-paying members; is affiliated with seventy-four lymphedema therapy centers; has an impressive medical advisory board that includes national and international experts; operates a toll-free support hotline; provides referrals to lymphedema treatment centers and health-care professionals; publishes a quarterly newsletter with information about medical and scientific developments, support groups, pen pals, and resources; conducts educational courses for health-care professionals and patients; and organizes an annual event called Lymphedema D-Day to honor inspirational lymphedema patients who have contributed to their communities or shown special courage in their struggle with the condition. The NLN has also sponsored national conferences on lymphedema. The first two of these gatherings attracted more than 500 participants from around the world.

Another example is that of Wendy Gelfand-Chaite. Wendy was a 32-year-old corporate litigator with a large law firm when she gave birth to her first child, Melanie. From the first year of her life, it was apparent that Melanie had lymphedema virtually throughout her entire body. Searching to understand the full nature of her daughter's condition, Wendy conducted exhaustive research but found only a limited body of knowledge about lymphedema and a demoralizing lack medical support. She herself performed manual lymph drainage for Melanie every day for three years until she was finally able to find a therapist whose treatment was covered by insurance and school-district funds. Because of the lack of medical options and the time commitment required to perform manual lymph drainage for her daughter, Wendy left her job and took a part-time position as a law professor. She sought information from every available resource, including top-notch children's hospitals throughout the country, lymphedema clinics, the National Organization of Rare Disorders (NORD), the NLN, and other parents of children with primary lymphedema.

One of the parents Wendy met was Dottie Morris. Dottie's young daughter Melissa had lymphedema in one leg, complicated by chronic cellulitis, despite her mother's meticulous care and rigorous applications of complex decongestive physiotherapy. Wendy and Dottie found comfort and support in sharing their experiences, frustrations, pain, and despair about the general lack of knowledge about congenital lymphedema. Together, they decided to turn their pain into power. With the support of NORD and the NLN, they established the Lymphedema Medical Project (LMP) and the Primary Lymphedema Action Network (PLAN). They assembled a multidisciplinary team of doctors, researchers, geneticists, clinicians, and members of the National Institutes of Health to lobby for greater medical and scientific research and funding, insurance reform, widespread lymphedema awareness and education, attention to the issue of lymphedema in medical schools, the development and recognition of lymphology as a medical specialty, and extensive media coverage of the condition. Informally, they refer to themselves as MOMS—Mothers With a Mission.

Yet another example of the power of individual action comes from Ann Fonfa, a breast-cancer survivor and member of SHARE (a national organization for breast- and ovarian-cancer patients) who is also a lymphedema patient and a self-educated expert who has written about lymphedema. In February of 1998, a three-day workshop entitled Lymphedema Forum was held in New York City. Sponsored by the American Cancer Society, the forum was attended by hundreds of doctors, nurses, political figures, lymphedema therapists, and lymphedema patients, among them doctors Robert Lerner, Jeanne Petrek, and Judith Casley-Smith, leaders in the lymphedema movement. The agenda for the workshop seemed to include everything one could dream of as far as hope for today and possibly a cure for the future: the epidemiology of the condition, treatment resources, current approaches to therapy, the list went on. Ann was scheduled to speak at the forum. However, when she received the agenda, she didn't like it. So she took action!

In a considered and well-phrased letter to the powers that be, she expressed her concern that those who actually suffered from lymphedema were not included in the forum's main discussions, which were to feature only physicians. She also noticed the absence of a focus on prevention. In her letter, Ann pointed out that the National Cancer Institute, and much of the National Institutes of Health, had recognized the value of lymphedema patients' perspectives and contributions. Further, she noted, having lymphedema patients contribute their input about such issues as sentinel-node biopsy (see page 23) might, in fact, spur on this protocol and thus reduce the incidence of lymphedema.

While Ann received widespread support from the doctors, clinicians, and researchers who were present, the ACS—which typically monitors and edits what people say at such forums—remained unyielding, excluding from the two-day discussion not only Ann but also Saskia Thiadens and other prominent therapists and impassioned patients. Nevertheless, Ann's actions set the stage for a power struggle that is sure to gain momentum as lymphedema therapists and patients—the true experts in lymphedema therapy—fight for a seat at the policy table. This kind of battle has been waged before, most notably by people with AIDS and breast-cancer survivors who have insisted, with great success, on being major players in the decisions, treatments, and policies that affect their very lives.

So what can *you* do? Quite simply, a lot! The first thing you can do is spread the word. Inform your doctor that all at-risk people need to be told, first, that they are at risk, and second, what they can do to prevent lymphedema from developing. This will be accomplished only when every single person facing lymph-node removal (for either diagnostic or treatment purposes) is informed by his or her physician that the removal of lymph nodes and the possible destruction of lymphatic vessels are predisposing factors for the condition. This doesn't mean just being told verbally. Any physician who treats trauma cases or performs surgery or radiation therapy should provide his or her patients with a written list of both preventive and treatment strategies. If your doctor says he or she is unaware of such strategies, this is the time when you can be your own impassioned advocate and your doctor's best resource. How?

• Share the relevant pages of this book with your physician.

• If you have already found a lymphedema center or a lymphedema therapist, have the specialist call your doctor (or have your doctor call the specialist). Doctors want to learn of effective treatments for lymphedema. Once they do, they become referral resources for other patients.

In addition, if your local hospital does not have a pink-wristband policy (see page 32), visit, call, or write to the chief executive and the nursing administrator and urge them to adopt one. Encourage them to issue the band routinely, as part of the admissions procedure; to stock pink wristbands in all departments at all times; and to train staff in the use and significance of the band. Suggest that emergency-room personnel include patients' lymphedema status on their questionnaires and, if it is determined that an emergency-room patient has or is at risk for lymphedema, that a pink band be placed on the patient's wrist immediately. Emergency-room patients are often seen by a variety of different medical personnel and sent to different departments for testing and other procedures. The pink wristband will serve to alert all concerned to a patient's status.

Additionally, ask that hospital personnel distribute literature about lymphedema to at-risk patients when they are discharged from the hospital. Too often, patients go home and engage in activities that increase their risk.

If your hospital declines to implement a pink-wristband policy, ask why. Contact the hospital administration again, especially the head of the nursing department. Explain that at-risk patients would be safer and more secure if affected limbs were properly identified. At the same time, encourage the hospital to make lymphedema therapy available. Point out that because of the rising incidence of this condition, no hospital—not even a small community hospital—should be without a special center, clinic, or unit devoted to lymphedema treatment.

Press the Issues

If you decide to become politically involved with the issue of lymphedema, or if you simply choose to speak about it with others, here are some of the pressing issues that will help people understand the condition better and know what must be done about it if progress is to be made:

• All medical and nursing schools should include courses about lymphedema, covering both prevention and treatment.

• All people who treat lymphedema should be trained and then certified or licensed by an expert doctor or lymphedema therapist who is already treating lymphedema patients. While the number of these practitioners is relatively small at this time, lymphedema therapy is such a specialized area that only they are equipped to judge the knowledge and skill of new practitioners.

• Those who treat lymphedema effectively, such as specially trained massage therapists, should be eligible for coverage under standard health-insurance policies.

• Legislation should be enacted to protect patients from abusive insurance-company practices such as withholding or denying payment for lymphedema therapy provided by those specially trained in the technique. And insurance companies should be required to ensure that patients have easy access to treatment.

• Congress should pass currently pending legislation requiring insurance companies to reimburse breast-cancer patients not only for surgery but for reconstruction, prostheses, and for any treatment indicated for "complications" of the surgery, including lymphedema. This bill (number S609 in the Senate and HR164 in the House of Representatives) is being cosponsored by Senator Edward Kennedy of Massachusetts and Representative Anna G. Eshoo of California.

• New research should be undertaken in the United States to find better and more effective treatments for lymphedema.

Some of the most significant social changes in history have come about because ordinary people have gotten angry or demoralized enough to echo the words of the besieged hero in the movie *Network*: "I'm mad as hell and I'm not going to take it anymore!" Spurred to action by the inequities of a system that seems more concerned with the bottom line than with the needs of the individual, they have gone public with their grievances, lobbied legislators for everything from wheelchair ramps to nonsmoking workplaces, and in so doing enhanced their own and other people's lives immeasurably. If and when you feel ready to do the same, you may find that your efforts have wide-reaching implications and that both you and society at large are better off for your efforts.

Spread the Word

Over the past several years, important treatments, policies, legislation, and studies have been brought about through the concerted efforts of breast-cancer and AIDS advocacy groups. The same is true of other conditions about which there was once little public awareness. If you are interested in making a difference in any of these areas as they relate to lymphedema, there are many ways to start, including talking up the issue:

• Engage in one-to-one communication, speaking with other people who have lymphedema about what you have learned, where you found beneficial treatment, or how you dealt with your insurance company, among other issues. This will empower them and possibly inspire them to speak to others.

• Join or start a lymphedema support group where you can discuss issues of concern on an ongoing basis.

• Participate in group and community education. Work with your local hospital to inform the institution's personnel of the importance of a lymphedema clinic and pink-wristband policy, or volunteer to speak to community groups about the importance of prevention, early treatment, and support for lymphedema patients.

• Write letters and petitions to your state health commissioner seeking a mandate for the use of the pink wristband in all hospitals.

• Start a letter-writing campaign to your local hospital that describes the importance of a legitimate lymphedema treatment center. Stressing legitimacy is important. Lymphedema patients do not need or deserve shoddy storefront centers staffed by untrained personnel. They need modern lymphedema centers staffed by professional therapists who are trained in and utilize the therapies known to be safest and achieve the best results.

• Conduct a letter-writing campaign to your elected officials on the federal level—your senators and member of the House of Representatives—pressing them to increase the amount of money the government allocates for research into the causes of, and effective treatments for, lymphedema. If the government can allocate money to study why people fall in love or why inmates want to escape from prison, it can certainly find the funds to investigate this lifelong condition![1] Inform your officials that you plan to tie the progress they make on this issue to your vote. To find the addresses and telephone and fax numbers of your U.S. representatives, call the U.S. Capitol Switchboard (see the Resources section at the end of the book).

• Conduct a similar letter-writing campaign to your state elected officials, urging them to take a leadership role in ensuring that insurance companies offer coverage for all effective treatments, as well as other insurance issues.

• Call the White House Opinion Line (see the Resources section at the end of the book) and tell the operator you are concerned about the lack of lymphedema research. Information about your call will be relayed to the President.

• Start a fund-raising project earmarked toward lymphedema research and let the local media know about your efforts.

• Become media-savvy. Make an appointment to see the editor of your local newspaper or the producer of a local television or radio show to suggest a feature or news story about lymphedema. Explain the importance and widespread nature of the condition and tell her or him your own first-person experience. Media people are always looking for topical stories that have relevance to their audiences.

• Write to breast-cancer and other special-interest health organizations and encourage them to publish information about lymphedema. The more publicity this condition receives, the better.

Before contacting anyone, be sure you have thoroughly researched the issues you plan to discuss and that you have the most current and accurate information. Always be as specific as possible, especially when asking about a particular research project or piece of legislation. Elected officials are interested in the hard facts that enable them to push legislation through. If you write or phone your legislators, or if you visit them personally, be sure to write a thank-you note afterward in which you restate your request. The more often you write, call, or visit, the more likely your expectations will be met.

However you choose to get involved, from stamping envelopes to participating in a support group to visiting a legislator to speaking publicly, the payoff will be priceless. As you begin to see the fruits of your labor taking shape, as you notice "the system" moving forward, even one millimeter at a time, you will know that your efforts made a difference—not only for yourself, but for the legions of people who have lymphedema and, better still, for those who may be able to avoid developing it in the first place.

GAIN CONTROL

Because the threat of medical malpractice suits has forced many doctors to practice defensive medicine, they will not suggest treatments that lie outside of their area of expertise or that are based on research from other countries. Consequently, people who are diagnosed even with diseases as common as breast or prostate cancer are often forced to do their own research into the best treatments, the newest therapies, and the most credible resources on which to base their decisions.

With lymphedema, unfortunately, this search is made more difficult because of the lack of publicity and scarcity of information. Many people don't even know where to begin. They are left with a disfigured limb, an increasing sense of isolation and despair and, in our blame-the-victim society, a growing feeling of self-contempt.

But in fact those who suffer from lymphedema are not alone. Experts say that one in eight American women will develop breast cancer at some point in her life, and it is estimated that 35 to 40 percent of women who undergo surgery for breast cancer develop lymphedema, at least to some degree.[2] Millions of people undergo other types of cancer surgery every year and millions more have serious accidents that damage their lymphatic systems. Most experts agree that about 10 percent of the people in these groups will get lymphedema as well.

By most accounts, the worst thing about illness is not knowing. Even in the face of the most frightening conditions, people often show amazing resilience *if* they know what is happening to them, what the condition entails, and what they can do to help themselves. The people who seem to combat disease most effectively are those who plunge into the activity of recovering, and the first step is knowing. Information is empowering. The better informed you are, the more knowledgeable your questions will be and the more in control, of both your life and your treatment, you will feel.

To take control in an otherwise uncontrollable situation, you must have the right tools. Luckily, in this age of information, those tools are available to everyone. They can be categorized under the tenacious acronym CLAW: call, look up, ask, write.

Call

The information you can get over your telephone is practically unlimited. All you need are the right questions and the kind of protocol that works well for investigative reporters, who make their livings by obtaining information. Again, using the journalist's Who?, What?, When?, Where?, Why?, How? format is useful.

You may be asking: "What can you tell me about [this drug, that treatment, et cetera]?" "When will I receive that information?" "Who is the author of that article?" "Why is this treatment recommended over another one?" "Where can I find. . . .?" "How does this [pump, compression garment, et cetera] actually work?" Here are some guidelines to help you become your own investigative reporter:

• Before you ask even one question, have a pen and pad of paper at your fingertips. For every call, be sure to write down your question, the date, the name of the person you speak to, where he or she is located, and, of course, the answer you receive. Keep this information in your lymphedema journal (see page 109) or in an easily accessible file so you can retrieve it when necessary.

• If your call has to be transferred to another extension, ask for that number so that you will be able to call back if you get disconnected.

• If you anticipate a complicated or lengthy answer, ask the person you are calling if it is all right for you to tape-record it. Most people who give out information over the phone feel comfortable about this if they are told ahead of time you will be taping. (You are also required by law to advise them of this.)

• Always identify yourself to the person who answers the phone, state your reason for calling, and ask if you have the right department. This simple introduction can save you a lot of time. And remember, the person who answers the telephone can be your best ally and point you in the right direction. The simple courtesy of a thank-you can go a long way in establishing good rapport.

• If you know the name of the place and the state from which you want information, call directory assistance. If you can't find local numbers in your telephone book, you can dial your local operator.

• Determine what you already know about the subject of your inquiry. If you are looking for information about a medication, you can narrow your search to your doctor; a local pharmacist, who may have literature on the drug in question; a medical library, where several reference books will have the desired information; or a knowledgeable friend.

• Once you learn the information is available, ask that it be mailed or faxed to you, or visit the library yourself to obtain it.

There are many individuals and organizations that are prepared to respond to telephone inquiries. ChemoCare is a valuable resource that allows you to speak with a pharmacist for information concerning drugs. For information about particular treatments, call your local medical library, the National Cancer Institute, or local cancer hotlines and support groups. (See the Resources section at the back of the book for further information.) Because cancer and lymphedema are so closely linked, cancer organizations can be good sources of information about lymphedema and its treatment. And, of course, among the best resources are your doctor and lymphedema therapist. Don't hesitate to call them.

In the recent past, increasing numbers of hospitals have set up lymphedema centers. Call the hospitals in your area to learn if such a center exists. If not, ask to speak to the hospital administrator and urge him or her to work toward the establishment of such a center. Many of the lymphedema centers that exist today were created as a result of information provided and pressure brought to bear by lymphedema patients themselves.

Look Up

If you are accustomed to visiting your local public library only to take out the latest bestseller, you may not be familiar with the vast resources many libraries offer, especially those affiliated with universities. Ask the reference librarian, who has special knowledge in accessing information from medical references, journals, and computer databases, for advice or help. Among thousands of library resources are computer databases found on Infotrac and books such as *Infomedicine: A Consumer's Guide to the Latest Medical Research*, by Fred Baldwin and Suzanne McInerney (Little Brown, 1996); *The Nutrition Bible*, by Barbara Deskins and Jean Anderson (William Morrow & Co., 1997); *Complete Drug Reference* (Consumer Reports Books, 1998); and *Alternative Health and Medicine Encyclopedia* (Gale Research, 1997).

Once you've found the book or article you're looking for—read, read, read! A good rule of thumb is to read medical books or medical and lay journals only if they were published within the last two or three years. With research and treatments changing literally by the day, it is important to be armed with the very latest information. This rule does not apply to first-person books about an author's own subjective experiences, however. Even if such a book is twenty years old, more often than not it will express feelings and offer insights that are just as powerful and affecting today as they were when they were written. First-person accounts can be both spiritually inspiring and pragmatically helpful.

Ask

"Here's some good advice: get good advice," is the sage advice offered by William Safire and Leonard Safir.[3] Good advice can be obtained from libraries, the Internet, and other sources, but sometimes a direct question posed to the right person is the most direct route to that much-desired answer.

Some people are inveterately curious. Whatever the subject, they want to know more about it and they don't hesitate to ask. Others may be just as curious, but shy about asking, fearing they will be intimidated by an expert or sound stupid or fail to formulate the perfect question.

If you are a person who hesitates to ask, try pretending that you are asking for important, even urgent, information about your child or pet. It's amazing how bold you can become on a loved one's behalf. Another strategy is to ask a family member or friend who has no qualms about asking questions to help you out. When faced with complicated conditions for which there are few treatments, people close to you often feel helpless. If you ask for their assistance with a specific task, most appreciate the opportunity to help and embrace it eagerly.

However you manage to ask questions, remember that you are doing so in the service of your health and your quality of life. If you succeed in gaining more knowledge—which you can then put into action—you will be better off, and so will your family, friends, associates, and even your pets, who will bask in your good feeling.

Write

If the telephone line is busy, the library far from your home, and a potential resource person not available, this is the time to rely on one of the world's oldest forms of communication—writing. In trying to gain information through writing, you should always write business-style letters. This requires a different form and style than a casual note or even a more formal personal letter:

• Make sure to include the name and title of the person you're writing to, the correct address and zip code, and the date of your correspondence.

- Before you write "Dear So-and-So," it is a good idea to include a line saying "Re: Lymphedema Treatment" (or whatever topic you're writing about).

- The first paragraph should include a brief personal introduction, summary of your situation, and your specific question. If you are requesting a copy of an article, abstract, monograph, or lecture, state its name, the author's name, and the date it was written (or delivered), or as much of this information as you know.

- Include a self-addressed stamped envelope (SASE) for the reply. If you are expecting anything of more than three or four pages, make sure the SASE has sufficient postage on it.

Writing can also be helpful on a more personal level. You may join a support group and find you cannot attend regularly because of physical limitations. If you have already established some friendships, you can correspond with your new friends to keep in touch and learn new information. Conversely, if someone else cannot attend, you can keep him or her apprised of the meeting's goings-on through writing.

CLAWing in Cyberspace

With the advent of the computer age, you can now write, call, ask, and look up all at one time if you have a computer with a modem and subscribe to an on-line service such as Prodigy, America Online, or CompuServe. Many people prefer the anonymity of computer correspondence and feel freer to share personal stories and exchange resources.

Through the Internet, which connects many thousands of computers worldwide, you can post messages and receive information from e-mail (electronic mail), computer bulletin boards, and from sites on the World Wide Web. People who communicate by computer learn of new literature, untested but effective treatments, medications, research, and even "cures," and often bring this information to their doctors.[4] If you have not yet entered the information superhighway, think seriously about taking a course in Internet communication. Or contact your local public library, hospital, or health-care provider to see if any of them have computers that can be used by the public. One word of caution, though: Anyone can post virtually anything on the Internet; the fact that something appears there is no guarantee that the information is accurate. Always check out the source of information before you act on it, as you would for anything you learned through word of mouth.

If your computer has a CD-ROM drive, you can use compact discs to do medical research or keep track of your medical records. Having a computer with a fax modem will enable you to receive information by fax as well as on-line. If you do not have a fax modem, you might want to consider buying a separate fax machine so that you can receive information in seconds.

Whichever way or ways of communicating you choose—choose! The more you learn and the more you know, the better able you will be to participate in your own treatment.

Conclusion

Before being diagnosed with lymphedema, many people spend years suffering with its symptoms, being told there is nothing they can do, or trying anything—elevation, cover-up clothing, self-help strategies—they hope will bring relief. As their symptoms get worse, they may feel increasingly isolated and depressed, and wonder why the great advances in modern medicine are unable to help them.

Well, as you now know, you are not alone. Millions of people suffer from this condition and, increasingly, they are being helped. You can be helped, too. The key to getting help is to make yourself as knowledgeable as possible about lymphedema, to become an active participant in your own health care, to collaborate with your doctor, and to seek out—today!—complete decongestive physiotherapy.

We have discussed the numerous ways that lymphedema patients can get the help they deserve. These strategies work. Read everything. Join a support group or start your own. Make your loved ones and coworkers aware of your condition and the ways in which they might help you. Bring the need for lymphedema care to the attention of your local hospital, encouraging them to open a lymphedema center and institute a pink-wristband policy. And get involved in bringing the pressing issues of lymphedema to the attention of your legislators, your insurance company, and the media.

Above all, don't despair. Increasingly, research institutions are studying ways to improve the diagnosis and treatment of lymphedema. While it is true that science often appears to progress at a snail's pace, significant progress has, in fact, been made in research related to the lymphatic system and lymphedema. In 1993, the International Congress of Lymphology met in Washington, DC, at a three-day conference entitled Frontiers in Lymphology. Two hundred seventy-five research papers were delivered by a group of international scientists with specialties in the vascular system and its disorders. In 1994, the National Lymphedema Network held its first conference, entitled Lymph Status: A Decade of Progress, in San Francisco, with 289 health-care professionals and patients presenting scientific papers and discussing numerous physiological, psychological, and treatment issues. The attendees came from Germany, Holland, Austria, Poland, the United Kingdom, New Zealand, Italy, France, Australia, and the United States. In 1996, the organization held its second national conference, Lymphedema: The Problem and the Challenge, in San Francisco, with hundreds of physicians, nurses, physical therapists, occupational therapists, massage therapists, and patients in attendance.

At all these conferences, research was presented that promises hope to people with lymphedema. While this body of work is encouraging, it does not include research on the psychosocial aspects of the condition—specifically, the effect lymphedema has on self-esteem and the degree to which it has an impact on every aspect of daily life.

Nevertheless, it is clear that current investigation is encouraging the scientific and medical communities to rethink many diagnostic and treatment methods that have changed very little in decades. It remains the challenge of lymphedema patients to stay on top of the latest research, the better to obtain the most accurate diagnoses and the best treatments possible.

Among research projects currently underway is a study to look at both invasive and noninvasive imaging techniques and the degree to which they can predict early cancers.[1] If cancer can be caught early, the extent of surgery can be minimized. Other current studies are assessing the effectiveness of sequential pumps, complete decongestive physiotherapy, manual lymph drainage and maintenance, and microsurgery for people with chronic lymphedema of the arm or leg.[2]

In addition, some researchers are now asking the question: Should the practice of removing and dissecting underarm lymph nodes of breast-cancer patients become extinct?[3] Others are exploring ways of altering the practice so that it is no longer necessary to remove more than one node.[4] (*See* Rethinking Lymph-Node Removal, page 23.) Since 182,000 women each year have breast cancer surgery in the United States, and 35 percent of them develop lymphedema at some time after surgery, the implications of this work are obvious.

Additional research is being done at the Stanford Lymphedema Center, where the Reid sleeve (see page 55) was developed. Basic research on lymphangiogenesis (the growth of new lymphatic vessels) being conducted under the direction of the center's director and former Harvard professor John P. Cooke, MD, may lead to the development of new, cutting-edge therapies to replace the vessels that are blocked in lymphedema. There are certain proteins that act to stimulate the growth of blood vessels; by administering these proteins, researchers hope to treat a number of different diseases characterized by blocked vessels, including not only lymphedema but coronary artery disease and peripheral vascular (blood-vessel) disease of the leg.

The causes and treatment of primary lymphedema are being studied as well. Mansoor Sarfarazi, PhD, a professor of human genetics and director of the Molecular Ophthalmic Genetics Laboratory at the University of Connecticut, together with his colleagues at the University of Connecticut Health Center, is conducting a study known as the Molecular Genetics Study of Lymphedema. They have found that certain types of lymphedema are inherited through multiple generations. In short, genetics plays a significant role in determining the risk that exists for children of people who are affected by lymphedema. The researchers are studying the entire genome—a person's entire genetic inheritance—of members of families in which lymphedema appears. Their goal is to identify a specific region on one of the twenty-two chromosomes that is shared by all (or at least most) of the affected members of the families under investigation. This technique, called positional mapping, seeks to find the gene or genes that give rise to inherited lymphedema, and the hope is that once the normal and abnormal functioning of the gene(s) responsible are fully investigated, it may be possible to to predict the risk of transmitting lymphedema to the next generation and also to develop some type of approach—medical, drug and/or gene therapy—to treat or cure it.

The study involves a group of families with different forms of lymphedema, using DNA (the ultimate genetic code) of both affected and unaffected family members. The researchers have identified several promising locations for the lymphedema gene and are recruiting additional families for the study with the aim of confirming one or more of the newly identified genes. Of course, the pace of good science is slow, so it may take many years of intensive research to obtain meaningful practical results.

Similar research is being conducted at the University of Pittsburgh by a team headed by David Finegold, MD, and Robert Ferrell, PhD. The goal of this project is to identify the gene or genes responsible for primary lymphedema in order to gain insight into its treatment and contribute to early identification of individuals at risk. Other research is being conducted by the husband-and- wife team of Marlys Witte, MD, and Charles Witte, MD, both professors of surgery at the University of Arizona College of Medicine. The founding directors of the Comprehensive Lymphedema-Angiodysplasia Diagnostic and Treatment Center at the Arizona Health Sciences Center/HealthSouth Rehabilitation Institute of Tucson, the Wittes evaluate and treat congenital lymphedema and acquired disorders of lymphatic circulation. Their research is multifaceted and includes, among other things, the study of lymphatic and blood-vessel formation; genes that are involved in familial lymphedema syndromes; the biology of lymphatic tissue and the causes, processes, development, and consequences of lymphatic-tissue disease; imaging techniques useful in evaluating the functioning of the lymphatic system; and therapeutic approaches that can enhance or reduce (as necessary) the proliferation of lymphatic and blood vessels. All of these studies on hereditary lymphedema welcome appropriate candidates (see the Resources section in the back of the book for additional information).

In addition to progress in research, doctors are becoming more aware of and sensitive to lymphedema, qualified lymphedema therapists are growing in numbers, lymphedema centers are proliferating, and networks of lymphedema patients are getting together to place this long-neglected condition on the map. All of these developments are helping people with lymphedema to get accurate diagnoses and, most important of all, the treatment they need.

We have spelled out a variety of strategies that may allow you to prevent the condition altogether if you should become a candidate for the kind of surgery or follow-up treatment that may place you at risk for lymphedema. By all means, utilize these strategies and share them with everyone you know who is facing surgery or radiation therapy. Unfortunately, it is also true that you can do everything right and still get lymphedema. If this happens to you, don't hesitate to seek aggressive treatment and learn how to manage the condition throughout your life.

With the conviction that you deserve the best treatment now available, you can make a difference in your own life and the lives of others who suffer from lymphedema.

References

Part I
Lymphedema: An Overview

Chapter 1
What is Lymphedema?

1. Judith R. Casley-Smith, PhD, MA, and J.R. Casley-Smith, DSc, MD, MBBS, *Information about Lymphoedema for Patients* (Adelaide, Australia: The Lymphoedema Association of Australia, 1995).

Saskia R.J. Thiadens, RN, "Lymphedema: An Information Booklet," 3rd ed., (San Francisco, CA: National Lymphedema Network, 1993).

2. I.H.M. Borel and A.B. deJongste, "Lymphangiosarcoma in Chronic Lymphedema. Reports of Three Cases and Review of the Literature," *Acta Chirurgica Scandinavica* 152 (March 1986): 227–30.

Chapter 2
Who Is Vulnerable to Lymphedema?

1. Sharon Batt, *Patient No More: The Politics of Breast Cancer* (Charlottetown, PEI, Canada: Gynergy Books, 1994), 332.

2. Marvin Boris, MD, Stanley Weindorf, MD, Bonnie Lasinski, MA, PT, and Gayle Boris, MD, "Lymphedema Reduction by Noninvasive Complex Lymphedema Therapy," *Oncology* Vol. 8, No.9 (September 1994), 95–106.

3. Jeanne A. Petrek, MD, and Robert Lerner, MD, "Lymphedema." In *Diseases of the Breast*, ed. Jay R. Harris, MD, Samuel Hellman, MD, and Monica Morrow, MD (New York, NY: J.B. Lippincott Co., 1996), 896–903.

4. Jeanne A. Petrek, MD, and Robert Lerner, MD, "Lymphedema."

5. Robert M. Kradjian, *Save Your Life from Breast Cancer* (New York: Berkley Publishing Group, 1994).

6. Marvin Boris, MD, Stanley Weindorf, MD, Bonnie Lasinski, MA, PT, and Gayle Boris, MD, "Lymphedema Reduction by Noninvasive Complex Lymphedema Therapy."

7. Michael W. DeGregorio and Valerie J. Wiebe, *Tamoxifen & Breast\Cancer* (New Haven, CT: Yale University Press, 1994), 45–51.

Inset: *Rethinking Lymph-Node Removal*

1. Robert M. Kradjian, *Save Your Life from Breast Cancer* (New York, NY: Berkley Publishing Group, 1994).
2. Richard G. Margolese, MD, Professor of Surgical Oncology, McGill University, excerpts from a panel discussion, "Problems in Management of Carcinoma of the Breast: Controversies, Problems, and Techniques in Surgery," Grand Hyatt Hotel, New York, NY, 9–11 December 1992.
3. Peter J. Deckers, MD, Chair, Department of Surgery, University of Connecticut School of Medicine, excerpts from a panel discussion, "Problems in Management of Carcinoma of the Breast: Controversies, Problems, and Techniques in Surgery," Grand Hyatt Hotel, New York, NY, 9–11 December 1992.
4. Rene Khafif, MD, Director of Surgical Oncology, Maimonides Medical Center, Brooklyn, New York, personal communication, December 1995.

**Part II
Treatment**

Introduction

1. Robert Lerner, M.D, "Lymphedema," pamphlet (New York, NY: Lymphedema Services, PC, 1993).
    Barbara J Carter, DNSc, RN, CS, "Psychosocial Aspects of Lymphedema," *National Lymphedema Network Newsletter* Vol. 7 No. 1 (January 1995), 4.

**Chapter 3
*Conventional Treatment***

1. Judith R. Casley-Smith, PhD, MA, and J.R. Casley-Smith, DSc, MD, MBBS, *Information about Lymphoedema for Patients* (Adelaide, Australia: The Lymphedema Association of Australia, Inc., 1995).
2. John R. Casley-Smith, DSc, MD. Marvin Boris, MD, Bonnie B. Lasinski, MA, PT, and Judith R. Casley-Smith, PhD, MA, "The Dangers of Using Pumps for the Treatment of Lympedema," paper delivered at the fifteenth International Congress of Lymphology, Sao Paulo-Recife, Brazil, 25–30 September 1995.
3. Ibid.
4. Ethel Földi, MD, and M. Földi, M.D, "Conservative Treatment of Lymphoedema of the Limbs," *Journal of Vascular Diseases* 35 (March 1995): 171–180.
5. Judith R. Casley-Smith, PhD, MA, and J.R. Casley-Smith, DSc, MD, "Volume Alterations in Lymphoedema; Untreated and After Complex Physical Therapy, Benzopyrones, or Both," *Newsletter of the XIV International Congress of Lymphology*, Washington, DC , September 1993, 35.
6. Marvin Boris, MD, Stanley Weindorf, MD, and Bonnie Lasinski, PT, "Persistence of Lymphedema Reduction After Noninvasive Complex Lyphedema Therapy," *Oncology* Vol. 11 No. 1 (1997): 99–109.
7. Iwona Swedborg, Jan-Richard Norrefalk, Neil B. Piller, and Christina Asard. "Lympoedema Post-Mastectomy: Is Elevation

Alone An Effective Treatment?" *Scandinavian Journal of Rehabilitation Medicine*, 25 (1993): 79–82.

8. Margaret Farncombe, MD, Gail Daniels, RPT, and Lisa Cross, MD, "Lymphedema: The Seemingly Forgotten Complication," *Journal of Pain and Symptom Management* Vol. 9 No. 4 (May 1994): 269–276.

9. Judith Casley-Smith, PhD, and John Casley-Smith, MD, "The Benzopyrones and Lymphedema," *National Lymphedema Network Newsletter,* January 1994: 1, 6.

10. Charles L. Loprinzi, MD, Mayo Clinic, Rochester, Minnesota, personal communication, March 1998. In this trial, women with chronic and prominent arm lymphedema were given either coumarin or a placebo for six months; after that time, the coumarin group began receiving an identical-appearing placebo and the placebo group began receiving coumarin. The women were checked at six and twelve months by means of arm measurement and patient questionnaires. Preliminary results indicated no substantial benefit from coumarin treatment.

11. Robert Lerner, MD, "Complete Decongestive Physiotherapy—An Innovative and Logical Approach to Lymphedema: Guidelines for Physicians and Patients," booklet (New York, NY: Lymphedema Services, PC, 1993).

12. V.M. Nava and W.T. Lawrence, "Liposuction on a Lymphedematous Arm," *Annals of Plastic Surgery* 21(4) (October 1988): 366–368.

13. M. Landthaler, U. Hohenleutner, and O. Bruan-Falco, "Acquired Lymphangioma of the Vulva: Palliative Treatment by Means of Laser Vaporization Carbon Dioxide," *Archives of Dermatology* Vol. 126 (July 1990): 967–968.

14. I. Katoh, K. Harada, Y. Tsuda, and others, "Intraarterial Lymphocytes Injection for Treatment of Lymphoedema," *Japanese Journal of Surgery* 14 (1984): 331–334.

15. K.R. Knight, M. Ritz, D.A. Lepore, R. Booth, K. Octigan, and B.M O'Brien, "Autologous Lymphocyte Therapy for Experimental Canine Lymphoedema: a Pilot Study," *Australian & New Zealand Journal of Surgery,* Vol. 64 No. 5 (May 1994): 332–337.

16. Cheryl I. Morgan, MSN, "A Comprehensive Approach to the Prevention and Treatment of Lymphostatic Ulcers," *National Lymphedema Network Newsletter,* July 1994, 1, 7.

Chapter 4
Alternative Treatments

1. O. Carl Simonton, MD, and Stephanie Simonton, PhD, *Getting Well Again* (Los Angeles, CA: J.P. Tarcher, 1978), 124–126.

2. Dan McGraw, "Flu Symptoms? Try Duck," *U.S. News & World Report,* 17 February 1997.

Chapter 5
Who Will Treat
Your Lymphedema?

1. Robert Lerner, M.D, "Lymphedema," pamphlet (New York, NY: Lymphedema Services, PC, 1993).

2. Interview format adapted from Judith R. Casley-Smith, PhD, MA,

and J.R. Casley-Smith, DSc, MD, MBBS, "How to Choose a Therapist," pamphlet (Adelaide, Australia: The Lymphedema Association of Australia, Inc., 1995).

Part III
Lifestyle Changes

Chapter 7
Diet and Exercise

1. A. Keys, *Coronary Heart Disease in Seven Countries,* Circulation 41 (Supplement 1) (1970): 211.
2. Walter Willet and Frank Sacks, "More On Chewing the Fat—The Good Fat and The Good Cholesterol" (editorial), *The New England Journal of Medicine* 325 (24): 1740.
3. Arlette J. Dinclaux, *Nutritherapy for Lymphedema* (Desert Hot Springs, CA: E.S.O.P. Publishing, 1995).
4. Cheryl I. Morgan, MSN, "A Comprehensive Approach to the Prevention and Treatment of Lymphostatic Ulcers," *National Lymphedema Network Newsletter,* July 1994: 1, 7.
5. Tina Adler, "Power Foods: Looking at How Nutrients May Fight Cancer," *Science News,* 22 April 1995.

Inset: *Natural Diuretics*

1. James F. Balch, MD, and Phyllis Balch, CNC, *Prescription for Nutritional Healing,* (Garden City Park, NY: Avery Publishing Group, 1990): 14, 225.

Michael Castleman, *The Healing Herbs* (Emmaus, PA: Rodale Press, 1991): 402.

Daniel B. Mowry, PhD, *The Scientific Validation of Herbal Medicine.* (New Canaan, CT: Keats Publishing, 1986), 81–84.

S. Taussig and S. Batkin, "Bromelain: The Enzyme Complex of Pineapple and its Clinical Application," *Ethnopharmacology* 22 (1988): 191–302.

Part IV
Dealing With Yourself and Others

Chapter 9
Your Emotions

1. Natalie Angier, "U.S. Opens the Door Just a Crack to Alternative Forms of Medicine," *The New York Times,* 10 January 1993, 1.

David Spiegel, MD, Joan Bloom, and others, "Effect of Psychosocial Treatment on Survival of Patients with Metastatic Breast Cancer," *Lancet* 2:8668 (14 October 1989): 888–891.
2. David Spiegel, MD, Joan Bloom, and others, "Effect of Psychosocial Treatment on Survival of Patients with Metastatic Breast Cancer."
3. Daniel Goleman, Ph.D., and Joel Gurin, eds., *Mind-Body Medicine: How to Use Your Mind for Better Health* (Yonkers, NY: Consumer Reports Books, 1993), 353–357.
4. O. Carl Simonton, MD, and Stephanie Simonton, PhD, *Getting Well Again* (Los Angeles, CA: J.P. Tarcher, 1978), 124–126.
5. Bernie Siegel, *Love, Medicine & Miracles* (New York, NY: Harper & Row, 1986), 24.

Chapter 11
Making a Difference

1. Former Senator William

Proxmire (D-WI) instituted what he called the Golden Fleece Awards to call attention to "wasteful, ridiculous or ironic use of the taxpayers' money." Among the winners: an $84,000 National Science Foundation study about why people fall in love; a $27,000 study to determine why inmates want to escape from prison; a $25,000 National Endowment for the Humanities grant to study why people cheat, lie, and act rudely on local Virginia tennis courts; a $219,592 Office of Education project to develop a curriculum to teach college students how to watch television; a $6,000, seventeen-page Army report instructing the federal government on how to buy a bottle of Worcestershire sauce. Just think of it—all these dubious subjects were deemed worthy of scientific inquiry, but not one cent was allocated to lymphedema research!

2. Ruby Bernstein, "Lymphedema Highlighted at Conference," *Breast Cancer Action Newsletter*, February 1995, 4.

3. William Safire and Leonard Safir, *Good Advice* (New York, NY: Times Books, 1982), xi.

4. William M. Bulkeley, "Untested Treatments, Cures, Find Stronghold on On-Line Services," *Wall Street Journal*, 27 February 1995, 1, A9.

Conclusion

1. A.P. Pecking, F.J. Bertrand, F.M. Likiec, J.H. Murray, M. Subramanian, A. Boudinet, J.L. Floiras, M.G. Hanna, Jr., and R.L. DeJager, Centre R. Huguenin, Saint-Cloud, France, and Organon Teknika/ Biotechnology Research Institute, Rockville, Maryland. "Preoperative Staging of Primary Breast Cancer by Immunolymphoscintigraphy," presentation at the International Congress of Lymphology, Washington, DC, September 1993.

E. Unger, Department of Radiology/MRI, University of Arizona College of Medicine, Tucson, Arizona. "Magnetic Resonance Imaging of Lymphatics and Lymph Nodes: Future Potential," presentation at the International Congress of Lymphology, Washington, DC, September 1993.

2. David M. Richmand, MD, Thomas F. O'Donnell, Jr., MD, Avigdor Zelikovski, MD, "Sequential Pneumatic Compression for Lymphedema: A Controlled Trial." *Archives of Surgery* Vol. 120 (October 1985).

M. Boris, MD, G. Boris, MD, and B. Lasinski, PT, Lymphedema Therapy, Woodbury, New York, "Initial Response to Complex Physical Therapy," presentation at the International Congress of Lymphology, Washington, DC, September 1993.

N.B. Piller, Red Cross Hospital, Stockholm, Sweden; I. Swedborg, Department of Primary Health Care, Flinders University of South Australia; N. Wilkingham Department of Oncology, Radiumhemmet, Stockholm, Sweden; and G. Jensen, Department of Oncology, Danderyds Hospital, Danderyd, Sweden, "Short-Term Manual Lymph Drainage Treatment and

Maintenance Therapy for Post-Mastectomy Lymphoedema," Presentation at the International Congress of Lymphology, Washington, DC, September 1993.

C. Campisi, J. Zattoni, C. Siani, and M. Casaccia, Department of General and Emergency Surgery, Microsurgery Center, University of Genoa; Department of Anesthesiology, University of Genoa, Genoa, Italy, "Twenty Year Clinical Experience in the Microsurgical Management of Lymphedema," presentation at the International Congress of Lymphology, Washington, DC, September 1993.

3. Peter J. Deckers, MD, Department of Surgery, University of Connecticut Health Center, Farmington, and Department of Surgery, Hartford Hospital, Hartford, Connecticut, "Axillary Dissection in Breast Cancer: When, Why, How Much, and for How Long? Another Operation Soon to be Extinct?" *Journal of Surgical Oncology*, 48 (1991): 217–219.

4. Rene Khafif, MD, Director of Surgical Oncology, Maimonides Medical Center, Brooklyn, New York, personal communication, December 1995.

Glossary

acupuncture. A type of treatment, based on traditional Chinese medical philosophy, that involves the insertion of extremely thin needles into the body at specific spots to relieve pain and treat illness.

adipose tissue. Connective tissue in the body that contains stored cellular fat.

adjuvant. A term used to describe auxiliary treatments, such as chemotherapy, radiation treatments, or hormone therapy, used after cancer surgery to help control, reduce, or destroy any microscopic collections of cancer cells that may have circulated to other parts of the body.

alternative treatment. Any type of treatment, including dietary regimens, herbal remedies, physical treatments, and meditative, spiritual, or religious treatments, that lie outside of the range of those recommended by conventional medical doctors. Also known as complementary or holistic medicine.

Americans With Disabilities Act. A federal law that guarantees equal opportunity in employment and equal access to public services, transportation, public accommodations, telecommunications services, and services provided by private entities. It protects anyone who has a physical and/or mental impairment that substantially limits his or her function in a "major life activity," such as caring for oneself, walking, seeing, hearing, speaking, breathing, learning, and/or working.

antibiotic. A drug or other substance that destroys or inhibits the growth of microorganisms.

axillary. Pertaining to or located in the area of the armpit.

axillary lymph-node dissection. A surgical procedure in which lymph nodes are removed from the underarm area.

benzopyrone. Any of a group of drugs that stimulate the body's immune system to help remove stagnant protein in tissue spaces. They are not approved by the Food and Drug Administration for routine use in the United States, but some doctors are using them on an experimental basis. Also called coumarins.

biofeedback. A technique that teaches a person to become aware of involuntary body functions (such as the beating of the heart or the regulation of body temperature or blood pressure), and to learn to control them by conscious effort.

biopsy. The removal of a small tissue sample for microscopic examination by a pathologist.

breast reconstruction. The creation of an artificial breast after mastectomy.

breast-conservation surgery. A surgical treatment for breast cancer in which the tumor, an area of normal tissue around it, and some axillary lymph nodes are removed. Other names for this type of surgery include lumpectomy, segmental mastectomy, and quadrantectomy.

cancer. A type of disease characterized by out-of-control, abnormal growth of cells that can invade and destroy healthy tissues. There are over 100 types of cancer. Also called malignant neoplasm or malignancy.

CAT scan. *See* Computerized axial tomography.

CDP. *See* Complete decongestive physiotherapy.

cellulitis. An infection of the soft tissues of the skin.

chemotherapy. Medical treatment using drugs. Cancer chemotherapy involves the use of highly toxic drugs, adminstered either orally or intravenously, that destroy cancer cells by interfering with their growth.

chiropractic. A system of health care based on the belief that disease is a result of misalignment of the spine, resulting in pressure on nerves that exit the spine to serve other parts of the body. Treatment involves manual manipulation of the spinal column and other body parts.

clinical trials. A procedure for evaluating possible new treatments conducted in human subjects after the treatment has demonstrated benefits in animal testing and in the laboratory setting. There are four phases of clinical trials: Phase I determines safe dosage and side effects. Phase II measures the effectiveness of the treatment. Phase III compares the treatment with the best known existing treatment. Phase IV establishes the new treatment as a standard therapy for patient use.

COBRA. *See* Consolidated Omnibus Budget Reconciliation Act.

collagen. A type of protein that is a key component of skin tissue.

color flow doppler test. An imaging test that utilizes ultrasound technology to create an image of the flow of fluids through the circulatory system and to detect any blockages.

complementary medicine. *See* Alternative treatment.

complete decongestive physiotherapy (CDP). An approach to treating lymphedema that combines decongestive therapy, treatment to break up areas of scarring, wrapping, and exercise.

compression garment. A sleeve or stocking that is a tightly knit one-piece elasticized-cotton garment, used to prevent fluid from flowing back and accumulating in a limb.

computerized axial tomography (CAT scan). A computerized x-ray examination that produces a highly detailed cross-sectional picture of the body.

congenital. Present from birth, but not necessary inherited.

Consolidated Omnibus Budget Reconciliation Act. A law under which you can continue your participation in an employer's group insurance plan for up to eighteen months after leaving your job by paying for it on your own. Known generally by its acronym, COBRA.

CT scan. *See* Computerized axial tomography.

decongestive therapy. Therapy that reduces the accumulation of fluid in the tissues.

dermatitis. Inflammation of the skin.

dermis. The middle layer of the skin. The dermis contains many of the skin's structures, including lymphatic vessels.

diagnosis. The process of determining the nature of a disease, which is a necessary preliminary to treatment.

diuretic. A drug or other substance that increases the output of urine.

edema. Swelling caused by the collection of fluid in the body's soft tissues.

edema, pitting. A term for edema in which small indentations, or pits, will form in the skin when it is pressed with a finger.

electrolytes. Mineral compounds that carry an electrical charge. They are the form in which vital minerals circulate in the body.

elephantiasis. A chronic condition, caused by obstruction of the lymphatic system, in which one or both of the legs become extremely enlarged and the skin and subcutaneous tissue become hardened.

endorphins. Chemicals produced in the brain that alleviate pain and elevate mood.

etiology. The cause of a disease.

extracellular fluid. Fluid found outside of individual cells. The extracellular fluid includes plasma, lymph, interstitial fluid, and transcellular fluid. Approximately one-third of the body's fluid is extracellular.

fibrosis. The formation of tissue in excess of amounts normally present; commonly referred to as scar tissue. Fibrotic tissue is harder than normal tissue.

guided imagery. A technique in which you help the healing process by visualizing mental pictures and images.

Halsted radical mastectomy. *See* Mastectomy, radical.

holistic medicine. *See* Alternative treatment.

homeopathy. A system of healing that utilizes remedies consisting of minute amounts of highly diluted natural substances to counteract specific symptoms of illness.

hormones. Specialized substances manufactured in several of the body's organs that travel through the bloodstream to stimulate activity in other organs.

hormonal therapy. Medical treatment that involves administering or blocking the action of certain hormones.

hyperkeratosis. A condition characterized by the appearance of patches of roughened skin.

immune system. The complex mechanism that defends and protects the body against bacterial, viral, and other invaders that threaten health and well-being. The lymphatic system is an important component of the immune system.

immunotherapy. Treatment directed at stimulating the body's immune system.

interstitial fluid. Fluid that surrounds and bathes the cells and is the source of lymph.

intracellular fluid. Fluid found within the body's cells. Approximately two-thirds of the body's fluid is intracellular.

intravenous (IV) infusion. A process by which fluids, glucose (sugar), electrolytes (soluble minerals), medications, or other substances are administered by means of a needle inserted into a vein. The needle is connected to a tube which in turn is connected to a bag of the solution(s) being administered.

iontophoresis. The introduction of soluble salt ions such as zinc oxide into the tissues by means of an electric current. Used as a treatment for lymphedematous ulcers, this increases blood flow and provides pain relief.

kinesiology. A treatment developed in the 1960s that involves the manual evaluation of the muscles and nerves in the body, and hands-on treatment to correct any imbalances.

LAS. *See* Lymphangioscintigraphy.

lesion. A localized area of abnormality of any tissue.

lipedema. A condition, seen primarily in women, in which abnormal deposits of adipose (fatty) tissue are found in the legs. It is characterized by grossly enlarged legs that bruise easily and are extremely sensitive to the touch.

liposuction. A surgical procedure in which fat is removed from selected areas of the body. It is sometimes used to debulk swollen lymphedematous limbs, as well as to treat lipedema.

Look Good—Feel Better. A program developed jointly by the American Cancer Society and the cosmetics industry to teach postmastectomy patients how to apply makeup and utilize scarves and turbans creatively to counteract the visible effects of chemotherapy and radiation and to boost self-esteem.

lumpectomy. *See* Breast-conservation surgery.

lymph. A clear, colorless body fluid composed of water, protein, salts, glucose, and urea, plus white blood cells. It originates in spaces in the tissues; when it enters the lymphatic vessels, it becomes known as lymph.

lymph node. Any of the small glands that remove wastes from the body's tissues and that contain infection-fighting white blood cells.

lymphadenitis. Inflammation of a lymph node.

lymphangioma. A benign tumor of lymphatic cells that develops in the lymphatic spaces and channels, resulting in an elevated skin lesion that may bleed, ooze, and become infected.

lymphangiosarcoma. A rare form of cancer affecting the tissues of the lymphatic system.

lymphangioscintigraphy (LAS). A test in which a radioactive solution is injected into the tissues and images are obtained as the radiotracer travels through the lymphatic system, creating detailed pictures of lymphatic channels and lymph nodes.

lymphangitis. A bacterial infection of the lymphatic channels.

lymphatic system. Part of the circulatory system, made up of nodes, vessels, and fluid. It is responsible for returning excess fluid from the tissues to the blood circulation, and also plays an important role in protecting the body against illness.

lymphatic vessels. Conduits through which lymph is moved through the body.

lymphedema. A chronic disorder in which lymph, a natural body fluid, fails to circulate properly and, as a result, accumulates in the tissues of a limb or other part of the body.

lymphedema, acute. Lymphedema that arises suddenly and lasts from three to six months.

lymphedema, chronic. Lymphedema that is not alleviated by elevation of the affected limb and that lasts longer than six months.

lymphedema, primary. Lympedema that is unrelated to any other known condition. Its cause is unknown.

lymphedema, secondary. Lymphedema that occurs following removal of lymph nodes or other damage to the lymphatic system, such as from radiation treatment or trauma.

lymphedema congenita. Primary lymphedema that is present from birth. Also known as Milroy's disease.

lymphedema praecox. Primary lymphedema that develops during adolescence or early adulthood.

lymphedema tarda. Primary lymphedema that develops during adulthood.

lymphocyte. A type of white blood cell formed in lymphatic tissue that is a vital constituent of the immune system. Lymphocytes fight infection and promote wound healing.

lymphology. The study of the lymphatic system and its disorders.

lymphotome. The area of the body that is drained by a particular lymph node or group of lymph nodes.

magnetic resonance imaging (MRI). A technique using powerful electromagnets, frequency waves, and a computer to diagnose and evaluate disease. It can be used to detect enlarged lymph nodes and abnormalities of the circulatory system, and to determine the extent of underlying tissue damage.

malignant. Literally, "evil." A term used to describe cancerous conditions.

manual lymph drainage (MLD). A type of rhythmic, segmental massage therapy used to treat lymphedema.

mastectomy. A surgical treatment for breast cancer in which all of the breast tissue and some of the lymph nodes in the armpits are removed. Also known as modified radical mastectomy.

mastectomy, radical. A surgical treatment for breast cancer in which the entire breast, the muscles of the chest wall, a portion of the surrounding skin, and all of the lymph nodes under the arm on that side are removed. Sometimes skin from another part of the body is required for a skin graft to the area. Also known as Halsted radical mastectomy.

mastectomy, segmental. *See* Breast-conservation surgery.

mediport. A device that is surgically implanted into the chest or arm with a temporary plug to accept an intravenous line.

melanoma. A systemic form of skin cancer that arises from a dark-pigmented malignant tumor.

metastasis. The spread of cancer cells from one location to another, usually through the bloodstream or lymphatic channels.

Milroy's disease. *See* Lymphedema congenita.

MLD. *See* Manual lymph drainage.

modified radical mastectomy. *See* Mastectomy.

MRI. *See* Magnetic resonance imaging.

oncology. The study of cancer and its treatments.

ordinary edema. *See* Edema.

osteopathy. A type of treatment in which hands-on manipulative techniques are used to treat illness.

physiatry. A medical specialty that focuses on physical and rehabilitative medicine.

pitting edema. *See* Edema, pitting.

plasma. The liquid portion of the blood.

platelets. Solid elements in the blood that help the blood to clot.

prosthesis. An artificial body form that replaces a missing body part.

protocol. The course of a particular treatment.

psychoneuroimmunology. The study of the interrelationships among the mind, the nervous system, and the immune system.

quadrantectomy. *See* breast-conservation surgery.

radiation therapy. A type of cancer treatment in which localized x-rays are aimed at a tumor and the immediate surrounding area to kill the cancerous cells.

radical mastectomy. *See* Mastectomy, radical.

red blood cells. Blood cells that carry oxygen from the lungs to the tissues throughout the body.

scrotum. The external sac of skin that surrounds the testicles.

segmental mastectomy. *See* Breast-conservation surgery.

sonogram. *See* Ultrasound.

steroid. A drug that is a synthetic version of the adrenal hormone cortisone, used to reduce inflammation. Steroids are powerful drugs whose side effects can include depression of immune function, fluid retention, and mental depression.

subcutaneous. Located just beneath the skin.

tamoxifen (Nolvadex). A drug that blocks the action of estrogen. It is used to treat certain types of breast cancer.

thymus. A small lymphatic organ located in the upper chest in which lymphocytes mature into T cells, a necessary component of the immune system.

transcellular fluid. Specialized extracellular fluids in the body that are separated from the interstitial fluid by membranes. Examples include cerebrospinal fluid, the fluid that lubricates the joints, digestive secretions, and the fluids in the eyes.

tumor. A group of cells or a mass that can be solid, semisolid (cystic), or inflammatory. Tumors may be malignant (cancerous) or benign.

ulcer. An inflamed sore that may lead to localized areas of tissue death. An ulcer can develop if an injury to the tissues goes untreated.

ultrasound. A type of technology used to create an image of soft tissue by bouncing sound waves off the part of the body to be studied. An ultrasound test may also be referred to as a sonogram.

white blood cell. Any of several types of infection-fighting cells that circulate in the blood. Some white blood cells are found in lymphatic tissue as well.

Resources

Listed in this section are sources of assistance with and information about lymphedema and related issues. Be aware that addresses and telephone numbers are subject to change.

In addition to organizations and practitioners, this list includes on-line services that provide support, encouragement, and other types of assistance beneficial to people with lymphedema. Here, too, be aware that addresses are subject to change, and that new resources are appearing all the time.

INFORMATION

Lymphedema

American Society of Lymphology
PO Box 14853
Lenexa, KS 66285-4853
E-mail: info@lymphology.com
Website: http://www.lymphology.com/
Provides information on lymphatic-system disorders and identifies health-care professionals and recognized treatment centers qualified to deliver recommended therapy.

Lymphedema International Network
E-mail: vda@gate.net
Website: http://www.lymphedema.com/
Internet resource that provides free information and education on the diagnosis and treatment of lymphedema plus various links to other sources.

Lymphoedema Association of Australia
94 Cambridge Terrace
SA 5061, Australia
61+(8) 8271–2198; fax 61+(8) 8271–8776
Email: casley@enternet.com.au
Website: http://www.lymphoedema.org.au/index.htm
Offers information and advice concerning lymphedema and its treatments.

Lymphovenous Canada
8 Silver Avenue
Toronto, ON M6R 1X8, Canada
(416) 533–2428; fax (416) 539–8348
E-mail: nermo@interlog.com
Website: http://www. interlog.com/~mcpherc/
*Links people in Canada who have lymphedema and other lymphatic-system
disorders to health-care professionals and support groups in their communities and around the world. Provides information on new research and
treatment.*

National Lymphatic and Venous Diseases Foundation, Inc.
255 Commandants Way
Chelsea, MA 02150
(800) 301–2103 or (617) 889–2103; fax (617) 887–1089
*Provides information about conditions of the venous and lymphatic systems
to medical and lay people.*

National Lymphedema Network
2211 Post Street, Suite 404
San Francisco, CA 94115-3427
(415) 921–1306; hotline (800) 541–3259; fax (415) 921–4284
E-mail: lymphnet@hooked.net
Website: http://www.hooked.net./~lymphnet
*Nonprofit membership organization that provides education and guidance
to patients, health-care professionals, and the public about the causes, symp-
toms, prevention, and management of primary and secondary lymphedema.
Membership includes a quarterly newsletter.*

Lymphedema Medical/Scientific Research Project
Wendy Chaite, Co-Coordinator
39 Pool Drive
Roslyn, NY 11576

(516) 625–9862; fax (516) 625–9410
E-mail lymphmom@aol.com
Dottie Morris, Co-Coordinator
72 Beacon Street
Melrose, MA 02176
(781) 662–1820; fax (781) 662–0451
E-mail: plandot@aol.com
Advocacy and interest group devoted to supporting medical and scientific research on primary and secondary lymphedema.

North American Vodder Association of Lymphatic Therapy
  (NAVALT)
1140 Turbin Road
Inman, SC 29349
(888) 4–NAVALT; fax (972) 243-3227
Network of Dr. Vodder School graduates who recommend lymphedema therapists throughout North America to people who have questions about lymphedema or may need treatment.

Northwest Lymphedema Center
1800 Northwest Market, Suite 203
Seattle, WA 98107
(206) 782–5598; fax (206) 782–2079
Nonprofit information and resource center that also sponsors a monthly lymphedema support-group meeting. JoAnn Rovig, the center's director, pioneered the self-care movement in the United States and developed two self-care videos that include information on the lymphatic system, manual lymph drainage, bandaging, compression garments, and the use of pumps. Profits from videos and donations go to help lymphedema patients who need financial assistance in buying garments and bandages.

Society of Vascular Medicine and Biology
Section of Vascular Medicine
University of Colorado School of Medicine
4200 East Ninth Avenue
Denver, CO 80262
(303) 270–4438; fax (303) 270–4037
E-mail: rajal002@maroon.tc.umn.edu
Website: http://www.svmb.org/lymph.htm
Offers an overview of lymphedema and links to various relevant sites.

Cancer

The American Cancer Society
1599 Clifton Road, NE
Atlanta, GA 30329
(800) ACS–2345
Website: http://www.cancer.org/cgi-bin/states.cgi
Answers general and specific questions about cancer, including causes, prevention, detection, treatment, and rehabilitation. Provides information on the programs and services, and refers people to their local ACS chapters.

American Foundation for Urologic Disease, Inc.
1128 North Charles Street
Baltimore, MD 21201
(410) 468–1800; fax (410) 468–1808
E-mail: admin@afud.org
Website: www.access.digex.net/~afud
Provides information about urologic diseases such as prostate cancer, as well as a support network.

Bosom Buddies Breast Cancer Support
776 Willow Brook Drive, No. 802
Naples, FL 34108–8541
(914) 514–3845; fax (941) 514–3846
E-mail: wsnobbie@juno.com
Website: http://www.go-icons.com/bosombuddies.htm
Offers ongoing education and support groups to women with breast cancer and lymphedema.

Cancer Information Service of Northern California and Nevada
32960 Alvarado-Niles Road, Suite 600
Union City, CA 94587
(510) 441–5793; fax (510) 475–1496
E-mail: mnaciona@nccc.org
Provides names and addresses of cancer centers that offer lymphedema treatment.

ChemoCare
231 North Avenue West
Westfield, NJ 07090

(908) 233–1103 (in New Jersey) or (800) 55–CHEMO (elsewhere);
    fax (908) 233–0228
E-mail: chemocare@aol.com
*A nonprofit organization that offers personal one-on-one support for people
undergoing chemotherapy and/or radiation treatment, provided by over 250
trained and certified volunteers who have survived the treatment themselves and understand the fears and concerns the patients encounter. Also
allows you to speak with a pharmacist for information concerning drugs.
Services are free and confidential.*

National Alliance of Breast Cancer Organizations (NABCO)
9 East 37th Street, 10th Floor
New York, NY 10016
(800) 719–9154
E-mail: NABCOinfo@aol.com
Website: http://www.nabco.org/
*Nonprofit resource for information about breast cancer: detection, treat-
ment, and possible related conditions such as lymphedema.*

National Breast Cancer Coalition
1707 L Street, NW, Suite 1060
Washington, D.C. 20036
(202) 296–7477; fax (202) 265–6854
E-mail: clhain@natlbcc.org
Website: http://www.natlbcc.org/
*Grassroots advocacy and resource group that focuses on research, preven-
tion, and finding a cure for breast cancer; encourages political involvement
with health issues related to breast cancer, including lymphedema.*

Prostate Cancer Survivor Support Group
US TOO International, Inc.
930 North York Road, Suite 50
Hinsdale, IL 60521-2993
(800) 808–7866 or (630) 323–1002; fax (630) 323–1003
Provides information about prostate cancer, as well as a support network.

SHARE (Self Help for Women with Breast or Ovarian Cancer)
19 West 44th Street, Suite 415
New York, NY 10036
(212) 719–0364; fax (212) 869–3431

English hotline (212) 382–2111; Spanish hotline (212) 719–4454
Lymphedema resource: Ann Fonfa
(212) 869–0139; E-mail Annfonfa@aol.com
Offers support and information for women with breast and ovarian cancer and lymphedema, as well as "A Consumer's View of Alternative Medicine" by Ann Fonfa, a book that covers treating lymphedema with alternative remedies.

Skin Cancer Foundation
245 Fifth Avenue, Suite 2402
New York, NY 10016
(212) 725–5176; fax (212) 725–5751
E-mail: info@skincancer.org
Website: http://www.skincancer.org
Provides information and referrals regarding all forms of skin cancer.

Y-ME National Breast Cancer Organization
212 West Van Buren, 5th Floor
Chicago, IL 60607-3907
(800) 221–2141
E-mail: help@y-me.org.
Website: http://www.y-me.org/index.html
Provides national hotline, support, resources, and information about cancer and related issues, including lymphedema.

General Medical Information

American Academy of Pain Management
13947 Mono Way #A
Sonora, CA 95370
(209) 533–9744
Offers free referrals to one or more of 6,000 certified practitioners who have degrees in dentistry, pharmacology, chiropractic, medicine, nursing, and/or physical therapy.

Health Resource Group
564 Locust Avenue
Conway, AK 72032
(501) 329–5272; fax (800) 329–9489
E-mail: moreinfo@thehealthresource.com

Website: http://www.thehealthresource.com
Offers mainstream and alternative/holistic treatment options for cancer and other conditions, information about specialists in various fields, and support organizations.

Knowledge Finder
Website: http://www.ariessys.com/
An electronic search system that gives you access to Medline, journals, databases, and other services.

Medicine OnLine
Foot of Broad Street
Stratford, CT 06497
(203) 375–7300; fax (203) 375–6699
E-mail: comcowic@meds.com
Website: http://www.meds.com
Offers medical information and education, literature searches, cancer discussion groups, and reading lists.

National Health Information Center
PO Box 1133
Washington, DC 20013–1133
(800) 336–4797
Provides a list of toll-free telephone numbers for information on health issues.

National Library of Medicine
8600 Rockville Pike
Bethesda, MD 20894
(888) 346–3656 or (301) 496–6308
Website: http://www.nlm.nih.gov
Provides free access to Medline's database of over 9 million references, abstracts, and journal articles.

National Organization for Rare Disorders (NORD)
PO Box 8923
New Fairfield, CT 06812-8923
(800) 999–6673; fax (203) 746–6481
E-mail: orphan@nord-rdb.com
Website: http: //www.nord-rdb.com/~orphan
A federation of more than 140 not-for-profit voluntary health organizations

dedicated to the treatment, prevention, and cure of rare ("orphan") diseases, including lymphedema.

PaperChase
Website: http://www.paperchase.com/
Path to Medline; provides access to medical literature.

Alternative Medicine (General)

Alternative Medicine Yellow Pages
1640 Tiburon Boulevard, Suite 2
Tiburon, CA 94920
(800) 333–HEAL
Offers a national directory of over 17,000 practitioners of alternative medicine, sorted by specialities, that may be purchased at bookstores or through the toll-free telephone number.

American Holistic Health Association
PO Box 17400
Anaheim, CA 92817
(714) 779–6152
E-mail: ahha.healthy.net
Website: healthy.net
A clearinghouse for free self-help resources promoting health and well-being.

American Holistic Medical Association
6728 Old McLean Village Drive
McLean, VA 22101
(703) 556–9728
Website: http://www.ahmaholistic.com
Offers a referral directory of specialists in holistic medicine

American Holistic Nurses Association
PO Box 2130
1733 East Lakin Drive, Suite 2
Flagstaff, AZ 86003-2130
(800) 278–AHNA or (520) 526–2196
Website: http://www.ahna.org
Offers alternative therapies in the home.

Foundation for Alternative Cancer Therapies (FACT)
PO Box 1242, Old Chelsea Station

New York, NY 10113
(212) 741–2790; fax (212) 924–3634
Nonprofit organization that offers referrals, resources, and guidance to cancer patients.

Foundation for the Advancement of Innovative Medicine (FAIM)
2 Executive Boulevard, Suite 404
Suffern, NY 10901
(914) 368–9797; fax (914) 368–0942
E-mail:faim@rockland.net
Website: http://www.healthworld.com/associations/chg/faim
  /index.html
Offers information and treatment of empirical clinical benefit that is outside the mainstream of conventional medicine.

Institute of Noetic Sciences
475 Gate Five Road, Suite 300
Sausalito, CA 94965
(415) 331–5650; fax (415) 331–5673
E-mail: Webmaster@noetic.org
Website: http://www.noetic.org/
Membership organization that encourages education on mediation, consciousness, human potential, and personal and social transformation. Has a quarterly magazine.

Office of Alternative Medicine
The National Institutes of Health Biological Medicine Institute
PO Box 8218
Silver Spring, MD 20907-8218
(888) 644–6226; fax (301) 495–4957
Website: http://www.altmed.od.nih.gov
Clearinghouse that distributes information regarding public inquiries of alternative mediciine.

Acupuncture

American Association of Oriental Medicine
433 Front Street
Catasauqua, PA 18032
(610) 266–1433; fax (610) 264–2768
E-mail: aaoml@aol.com

Website: http://www.aaom.org
Nationally certified practitioners of oriental medicine offer information, education, and serve as a resource for legislators and the general public regarding acupuncture and Oriental medicine. Offers free referrals to over 1,200 acupuncturist members who have completed training and passed a national certification exam, and are state licensed.

National Acupuncture and Oriental Medicine Alliance
14637 Starr Road SE
Olalla, WA 98359
Website: http://www.healthy.net/naoma
Offers free referrals from databases of 4,000 acupuncturists who are either state licensed or national board certified.

Biofeedback

Association for Applied Psychophysiology and Biofeedback
10200 West 44th Avenue, Suite 304
Wheat Ridge, CO 80033
(303) 422–8436
E-mail: aapb@resourcenter.com
Website: http://www.aapb.org
Offers informational pamphlet and list of practitioners throughout the country who specialize in pain management and stress reduction.

Biofeedback Certification Institute of America
10200 West 44th Avenue, Suite 304
Wheatridge, CO 80033
(303) 420–2902
Offers free referrals to over 1,500 practitioners who are trained and certified in various modalities of biofeedback therapy. Written requests only with enclosed starnped, self-addressed commercial-size (No. 10) envelope.

Chiropractic

American Chiropractic Association
1701 Clarendon Boulevard
Arlington, VA 22209
(703) 276–8800

Offers free referrals from 21,500 members who do spinal adjustment and medically oriented supplemental therapies. All are licensed doctors of chiropractic with over five years of postgraduate training and internship through accredited chiropractic colleges.

Guided Imagery

Academy for Guided Imagery
PO Box 2070
Mill Valley, CA 94942
(800) 726–2070
Offers books and tapes for lay people and professionals relating to the use of imagery in healing. Free catalog.

Simonton Cancer Center
PO Box 890
Pacific Palisades, CA 90272
(310) 459–4434; fax (310) 457–0421
E-mail: simonton@lainet.com
Offers residential program for cancer patients, as well as tapes and literature on guided imagery.

Herbal Medicine

American Botanical Council
PO Box 201660
Austin, TX 78720
(512) 331–8868; fax (512) 331–1924
E-mail: abc@herbalgram.org
Website: herbalgram.org
Offers educational books, videos, and software on responsible use of herbal medicines, and a quarterly magazine.

American Herbalists Guild
PO Box 746555
Arvada, CO 80006
(303) 423–8800; fax (303) 402–1564
E-mail: ahgoffice@earthlink.net
Provides literature and information about herbs and their uses. Offers free referrals to about 100 professional member herbalists approved by their peer-review board.

Wise Woman Center
PO Box 64
Woodstock, NY 12498
(914) 246–8081 (phone and fax)
Provides books, tapes, and classes on herbal medicine.

Homeopathy

Homeopathic Academy of Naturopathic Physicians
12132 SE Foster Place
Portland, OR 97266
(503) 761–3298
For a small fee, will provide a list of naturopathic physicians certified in classical homeopathy. All have completed at least 250 hours of study and at least one year of clinical experience.

Homeopathic Educational Services
2124 Kittredge Street
Berkeley, CA 94704
(800) 359–9051 or (510) 649–0294
Websites: http://www.homeopathy-request@lyghtforce.com
                    http://www.arnica.com
                    http://www.somtel.com/homeovernight/
Provides books and tapes and homecare kits.

International Foundation for Homeopathy
2366 Eastlake Avenue East, Suite 301
Seattle, WA 98102
(206) 324–8230
Provides educational courses.

National Center for Homeopathy
801 North Fairfax, Suite 306
Alexandria, VA 22314
(703) 548–7790
Provides referrals to practicing homeopaths.

Hypnotherapy

American Board of Hypnotherapy
16842 Von Karman Avenue, Suite 475
Irvine, CA 92606
(800) 634–9766; fax (714) 251–4632
E-mail: aih@ix.netcom.com
Website: http://www.hypnosis.com
Offers free referrals to 10,000 member hypnotherapists who have completed approved training, been certified and registered by ABH.

Massage

Nursing Touch and Massage Therapy Association
PO Box 1173
Abita Springs, LA 70420
(504) 892–6990
Offers free referrals to over 700 members. All are licensed nurses plus therapeutic touch and/or massage therapists.

Meditation

Institute of Transpersonal Psychology
PO Box 4437
Stanford, CA 94305
(415) 327–2066
Provides research information and referrals.

Mind-Body Health Sciences, Inc.
393 Dixon Road
Boulder, CO 80302
(303) 440–8460
Provides speakers on mind-body medicine and has books on meditation and music on tape.

Maharishi International University
1000 North 4th Street
Fairfield, IA 52556
(515) 472–5031
Provides literature about research in transcendental meditation.

Diet and Nutrition

American Academy of Nutrition
3408 Sausalito Drive
Corona Del Mar, CA 92625
(800) 290–4226
Offers free referrals to one or more of over 400 graduates of a fifteen-month comprehensive program offered by this home-study school of nutrition. Accredited by the Distance Education and Training Council of the U.S. Department of Education.

Mental Health

American Psychiatric Association
Division of Public Affairs
Department FXI
1400 K Street, NW
Washington, DC 20005
(202) 682–6000
Upon written request, offers free referrals to one or more of 39,000 certified psychiatrist members via district branch nearest you. Free pamphlets available on mental illness and choosing a psychiatrist.

American Psychological Association
750 First Street, NE
Washington, DC 20002
(800) 964–2000
Offers free referrals to over one or more of 60,000 members, who have PhDs in psychology or related fields. National office will refer you to a local association chapter in your state.

Support Group Information

American Self-Help Clearinghouse
Saint Clares-Riverside Medical Center
25 Pocono Road
Denville, NJ 07834
(201) 625–9565 or (201) 625–7101; fax (201) 625–8848
Website: http://www.reeusda.gov/pavnet/cf/cfamersh.htm
Tracks 700 different support groups throughout the country and publishes "The Self-Help Sourcebook," which offers advice on setting up your own support group.

Employment Issues

U.S. Equal Employment Opportunity Commission
1801 L Street, NW
Washington, DC 20507
(800) 669–4000 or (202) 663–4900
Website: http://www.eeoc.gov/
Enforces federal legislation prohibiting discrimination in employment.

Insurance Issues

Health Insurance Association of America
555 13th Street NW
Washington, DC 20004
(202) 824–1600
E-mail: webmaster@hiaa.org
Website: http://www.hiaa.org/
Provides guides for consumers on such subjects as disability income, health insurance, long-term care, and Medicare.

Advocacy

Congress.Org
Website: http://www.congress.org/
Offers access to a complete and reliable directory of information about the members of the U.S. House of Representatives and Senate.

Electronic Frontier Foundation
Website: http://www.eff.org/pub/Activism/Congress_contact/
Offers contact information and database archives on the U.S. Congress.

FedNet
Website: http://www.fednet.net/
Provides access to numerous facets of the U.S. government, including broadcast coverage of Congress, federal agencies, and the White House, and breaking news events in the nation's capital. Coverage provided is unedited and without commentary, providing an unfiltered view of the government at work.

Senate E-Mail List
Website: http://www.northernwebs.com/senate/
Offers a complete list of U.S. senators and their e-mail addresses.

U.S. Capitol Switchboard
(202) 224–3121
Will connect you directly with the office of any U.S. Senator or Representative you wish to contact.

U.S. Congress Handbook
Website: http://www.congress-handbook.com/
The U.S. Congress Handbook and related products offer quick access to information about our national legislature and its members.

U.S. House of Representatives.
Website: http://www.house.gov/
The website of the U.S. House of Representatives. Offers information about the House and its members, as well as a link to allow you to write to your representative.

Vote-Smart
Website: http://www.vote-smart.org/
Can provide address, telephone, fax, and e-mail information for federal elected representatives.

White House Opinion Line
(202) 456–1111
You can call this line to express your opinions about any issue(s) of concern; information about your call will be relayed to the President.

PRODUCTS

Compression Garments and Pumps

The following is a list of some of the many manufacturers and suppliers of pumps and compression garments in the United States. Many suppliers will help you measure and fit a compression garment and/or deliver the product to your home.

Barton-Carey Custom Stockings
PO Box 421
Perrysburg, OH 43552
(800) 421–0444; fax (419) 874–0888
Manufacturer of compression garments.

Beiersdorf, Inc. Bandages & Padding
BDF Plaza
Norwalk, CT 06856
(800) 876–3664, extension 805
Manufacturer of compression garments.

Beiersdorf-Jobst, Inc.
5825 Carnegie Boulevard
Charlotte, NC 28209
(704) 554–9933 or (704) 551–7189
Offers complete line of products for lymphedema management, including those for skin care, bandaging, and compression.

Bio Compression Sequential Circulator
120 West Commercial Avenue
Moonachie, NJ 07074
(800) 222–PUMP; fax (888) 663–3362
Manufacturer of pumps and mattresses.

The Care Group
2525 West Belfort, Suite 150
Houston, TX 77054
(800) 289–8001 or (800) 289–8025
Acts as a representative for manufacturers of lymphedema pumps (sells to physicians).

CBF
8044 Ray Mears Boulevard, Suite 100
Knoxville, TN 37919
(800) 225–8129
Supplier of compression garments and postmastectomy prostheses directly to patients.

CircAid Medical Products, Inc.
9323 Chesapeake Drive, Suite B-1
San Diego, CA 92123
(800) CIRCAID or (619) 576–3550; fax (619) 576–3555
E-mail:info@circaid.com
Website: http://www.circaid.com/index.html
Manufacturer of nonelastic, Velcro compression garments.

Compass Health Care, Inc.
3333 Vine Street, Suite 103
Cincinatti, OH 45220
(513) 961–3144; fax (513) 961–5070
Supplier of pumps and custom-made compression garments.

Day Drug & Surgical Company
1912 Deer Park Avenue
Deer Park, NY 11729
(516) 667–7880; fax (516) 242–0719
Supplier of pumps and made-to-order compression sleeves (doctor's prescription required).

Freeman Manufacturing Company
900 West Chicago Road
Sturgis, MI 49091
(616) 651–2371; fax (616) 651–8248
Manufacturer of compression garments in wide range of sizes and styles.

Innovative Medical Inc.
PO Box 101314
Birmingham, AL 35210
(205) 699–1887; fax (205) 629–7611
Supplier of pumps (doctor's prescription required).

J&C Associates, Inc
212 High Street
Geneva, NY 14456-2219
(800) 756–7269 or (315) 789–1822; fax (315) 781–2349
E-mail: jmarsh@jobst.net
Website: http://www.jobst.net
Certified fitter of Jobst compression products.

Jobst
Elvarex (Varitex-Beiersdorf)
Box 653
Toledo, OH 43697–0653
(800) 537–1063 or (419) 698–1611; fax (419) 691–4511
Manufacturer of compression garments that are very good. However, the range is not large and the sleeve will only fit a fairly bulky shoulder.

Jobst Service Center
4602 North 16th Street, Suite 305
Phoenix, AZ 85016
(602) 235–9130; fax (602) 235–9298
Manufacturer of bandages and custom-made compression garments. Offers delivery within seven to ten days.

Juzo (Julius Zorn Inc.)
PO Box 1088
80 Chart Road
Cuyahoga Falls, OH 44223
(800) 222–4999; fax (800) 645–2519
E-mail: support@juzousa.com (for general information)
          sales@juzousa.com (for dealer support)
Manufacturer of compresssion garments that come in a wide range of sizes and styles.

Legacy Directional Flow Compression System
1800 NW market, Suite 210
Seattle, WA 98107
(206) 782–8554
Supplier of a compression sleeve of padded foam to place under bandages or pump sleeve or to use in lieu of overnight bandaging. The sleeve, which is used in combination with an outside adjustable Velcro jacket, has pressure points that work on fibrotic deposits and direct the flow of lymph in same direction as does manual lymphatic drainage. The sleeve was developed by manual lymphatic therapist JoAnn Rovig and Donald Kellogg, the codeveloper of the Reid sleeve.

Medi Stockings & Sleeves
76 West Seegers Road
Arlington Heights, IL 60005
(800) 633–6334; fax (847) 640–0209
Manufacturer of compression garments and pantyhose.

Mego Afek
Kibbutz Afek 30042
Israel
972–4–8784277; fax 972–4–8784148
E-mail: megoafek@doryanet.co.il
Website: http://www.doryanet.co.il/megoafek/default.html

Develops and distributes medical devices worldwide, including pneumatic sequential compression, for lymphatic and venous disorders, including lymphedema.

Peninsula Medical
PO Box 7317
Stanford, CA 94309-7317
(800) 29–EDEMA
E-mail: edemarx@aol.com
Supplier of the Reid sleeve.

Perfect Fit, Inc.
1895 Post Road
Fairfield, CT 06430
(203) 255–0766; fax (203) 259–6620
Website: http://www.sbshow.com/CT/PerfectFit/default.html
Supplier of compression garments and pumps.

Prescription Devices, Inc.
99 NW 11th Street
Boca Raton, FL 33432
(800) 940–8989 or (561) 391–8989
Supplier of home medical equipment (doctor's prescription required).

Sigvaris (Ganzoni)
Box 570, 32 Park Drive East
Branford, CT 06405
(800) 322–7744; fax (203) 481–5488
Manufacturer of compression garments, including gloves, that come in a wide range of sizes and styles.

West Val Medical Supplies
5363 Balboa Boulevard, Suite 142
Encino, CA 91316
(818) 981–2600 or (818) 362–5011; fax (818) 981–3967
Supplier of compression garments and home medical equipment (doctor's prescription required).

Wright Linear Pumps, Inc.
303 Robinson Road

Imperial, PA 15126
(800) 631–9535; fax (724) 695–0406
Manufacturer of pumps.

Medications

The International Academy of Compounding Pharmacies
PO Box 365
Sugarland, TX 77487
(800) 927–4227; fax (281) 495–0602
E-mail: jwicker@iacprx.org
Website: http://www.iacprx.org
Can assist in locating a compounding pharmacy in your area that can prepare and supply benzopyrones (with a doctor's prescription, of course).

Other

Big Pine Birds
1501 East Prospect Lane
Tucson, AZ 85719
(520) 323–7953
E-mail: chivers@ag.arizona.edu
Supplier of emu oil to individuals.

Lymphedema Alert Bracelet
National Lymphedema Network
2211 Post Avenue, Suite 404
San Francisco, CA 94115–3427
(800) 541–3259; fax (415) 921–4284
Website: http://hooked.net/~lymphnet
Provides nonallergenic stainless-steel wristband.

MedicAlert
2323 Colorado Avenue
Turlock, CA 95382
(800) 432–5378
Provides bracelets and necklaces that contain personalized medical information and warn about chronic medical conditions.

Pink Wrist Band
c/o Diane Sackett Nannery
PO Box 699
Manorville, New York 11949–0669
Supplier of reusable, adjustable pink wristbands. All proceeds go to lymphedema research.

PROFESSIONAL SERVICES

Diagnostic and Treatment Centers and Manual Lymphatic Therapists

The following is a list of lymphedema diagnostic and treatment centers and practitioners by geographic area. For each area, facilities are listed first, followed by individual practioners. Please note this list is for information only and does not constitute an endorsement of any particular center or practitioner. Always ask about fees, and consult with your physician and follow the guidelines in this book to ensure that you are receiving safe and informed treatment. It is wise to verify that the treatments are covered by your insurance company before undergoing treatment.

The facilities listed here employ medical and/or other health-care professionals such as medical doctors (MDs), registered nurses (RNs), physical therapist (PTs), occupational therapists (OTs), or licensed massage therapists (LMTs). All certified lymphedema therapists mentioned here have, in addition to their other professional training, taken special training in manual lymph drainage (MLD) and complete decongestive physiotherapy (CDP). Wherever possible, the addresses of lymphedema therapists who practice independently have been included. Some therapists, however, preferred that their addresses not be listed. Please be aware that addresses and telephone numbers are subject to change.

Alaska

Alaska Alternative Medicine Center
3201 C Street, Suite 602
Anchorage, AK 99503
(907) 563–6200; fax (907) 561–4933
E-mail: aamc@servcom.com
Provides CDP/MLD by certified therapists.

Arizona

A Therapeutic Touch and Integrated Lymphatic Therapy
4491 North Cerritos Drive
Tucson, AZ 85745
(520) 743–8135; fax (520) 743–9326
E-mail: specialhands@juno.com
Provides CDP/MLD by certified therapists.

Nova Care Rehabilitation Institute of Tucson
6367 East Tanque Verde Road, Suite LL-10
Tuscon, AZ 85715
(520) 721–0319; fax (520) 721–2287
Provides CDP/MLD by certified therapists.

University of Arizona With HealthSouth Rehabilitation
  Institute of Tucson
Department of Surgery
PO Box 245063
Tucson, AZ 85724-5063
(520) 626–6118; fax (520) 626–0822
E-mail: lymph@u.dot.arizona.edu.
Provides a broad spectrum of diagnostic and treatment modalities for lymphedema patients, together with an extensive research program.

Susan Couture, LMT
4749 East San Francisco Boulevard
Tucson, AZ 85712
(520) 326–7702
E-mail: couture@azstarnet.com
Certified CDP/MLD therapist.

Sarah Ann Taylor, LMT
3139 North 40th Street, No. 4
Phoenix, AZ 85018
(602) 381–1904
Certified CDP/MLD therapist.

California

Aurora Lymphedema Clinic
2211 Post Street, Suite 404
San Francisco, CA 94115
(415) 921–2911 or (415) 921–4284
Provides CDP/MLD by certified therapists.

Beauty Kliniek
3268 Governor Drive
San Diego, CA 92122
(619) 457–0191; fax (619) 457–0378
Provides CDP/MLD by certified therapists.

Ginger-K Center
1202 Meridian Avenue
San Jose, CA 95125-5209
(408) 445–8626; fax (408) 723–3797
*Cancer treatment center that provides CDP/MLD by trained therapists.
Also has a twice-monthly support group.*

Healthline One
PO Box 230788
Encinitas, CA 92023
(800) 99–WORLD; fax (888) 596–7439
Provides pump therapy and compression-garment fitting and adjustment.

Hoag Memorial Hospital Presbyterian-Rehabilitation Services
Newport Beach, CA 92663
(714) 760–5645; fax (714) 760–5648
Provides CDP/MLD by certified therapists.

Mesa Physical Therapy Center
7510 Claremont-Mesa Blvd., Suite 103
San Diego, CA 92111
(619) 277–2277; fax (619) 277–7358
Provides CDP/MLD by certified therapists.

Mount Diablo Medical Center
Lymphedema Center/Physical Medicine Department

PO Box 4110
2540 East Street
Concord, CA 94524
(510) 674–2125; fax (510) 674–2378
Provides CDP/MLD by certified therapists.

Naval Medical Center Breast Health Center
34800 Bob Wilson Drive, Suite 207
San Diego, CA 92134–1207
(619) 532–5821 or (619) 532–5811
E-mail: tmondry@snd10.med.navy.mil
Provides CDP/MLD by certified therapists for Department of Defense health-care beneficiaries.

North State Lymphedema Center
274 Cohasset Road, Suite 110
Chico, CA 95926
(530) 891–6042; fax (530) 891–6374
Provides CDP/MLD by certified therapists.

Northern California Compression Therapy Center, Inc.
6611 Coyle Avenue
Carmichael, CA 95608
(916) 961–6800; fax (916) 961–2919
Provides CDP/MLD by certified therapists.

Primedical
969-G Edgewater Boulevard, Suite 392
Foster City, CA 94404
(650) 780–6795; fax (650) 574–9274
Provides CDP/MLD by certified therapists.

Queen of the Valley Hospital Physical Therapy Department
1000 Trancas Street
Napa, CA 94558
(707) 257–4089; fax (707) 257–4157
Provides CDP/MLD by certified therapists.

Redding Physical Therapy Center
1740 Eureka Way
Redding, CA 96001

(530) 243–1102; fax (530) 243–1123
Provides CDP/MLD by certified therapists.

Rehabilitation Institute of Santa Barbara Outpatient Center
2921 De La Vina
Santa Barbara, CA 93105
(805) 967–6631; fax (805) 569–2563
Provides CDP/MLD by certified therapists.

Stanford University Medical Center Division of
    Cardiovascular Medicine
300 Pasteur Drive
Stanford, CA 94305-5406
(415) 725–3778; fax (650) 725–1599
E-mail: john.cooke@forsyth.stanford.edu
Website: http://www-med.stanford.edu/school/lymphedema/
Provides a broad spectrum of diagnostic and treatment modalities for lymphedema patients, together with an extensive research program.

UCLA Medical Center Rehabilitation Services
300 UCLA Medical Plaza, Suite B-100
Los Angeles, CA 90095
(310) 794–1323; fax (310) 794–1457
Provides CDP/MLD by certified therapists.

Wyrick Institute and Clinic
PO Box 99745
San Diego, CA 92169
(619) 273–9764
Provides CDP/MLD by certified therapists.

Marchelle Brown
Santa Monica, CA
(310) 393–2173
Certified CDP/MLD therapist.

Mary P. Crane, OTR
2030 Viborg, Suite 118
Solvang, CA 93463
(805) 686-9316; fax (805) 688-2231
E-mail: mcplays@aol.com
Registered Occupational Therapist

Richelle Drake, LMT
16334 Moorpark Street
Encino, CA 91436
(818) 783–4579; fax (818) 783–6280
Certified CDP/MLD therapist.

Robert Kradjian, MD
1800 Sullivan Avenue, Suite 302
Daly City, CA 94015
(415) 343–2262; fax (415) 579–6040
Breast surgeon experienced in diagnosing lymphedema and recommending appropriate treatment.

Camille Newlon, PT
2560 Garden Road, No. 228
Monterey, CA 93940
(408) 656–0511; fax (408) 656–0535
Certified CDP/MLD therapist.

Patricia Wiltse, LMT
San Francisco, CA
(415) 776–4480; fax (415) 776–4480
Certified CDP/MLD therapist.

Colorado

Lutheran Medical Center Physical Medicine and
 Rehabilitation Department
8300 West 38th Avenue
Wheat Ridge, CO 80033
(303) 425–2425; fax (303) 467–8780
Provides CDP/MLD by trained therapists.

Lymphedema Center
8200 East Belleview
Central Tower
Englewood, CO 80111
(303) 741–0017; fax (303) 267–8294
Website: http://www.sjbnet.com
Provides evaluation and comprehensive treatment of lymphedema by certified therapists.

Vineeta Lovell, LMT
725 Mead Street, No. 3
Louisville, CO 80027
(303) 604–2911
Certified CDP/MLD therapist.

Connecticut

Connal Physical Therapy Group
6 Poquonock Avenue, Suite 11
Windsor, CT 06095
(860) 683–0080; fax (860) 683–2614
Website: http://www.cshore.com/connal
Provides CDP/MLD by certified therapists.

Easter Seals Rehabilitation Center
26 Palmer's Hill Road
Stamford, CT 06902
(203) 325–1544; fax (203) 327–5135
Provides CDP/MLD by certified therapists.

Main Street Physical Rehabilitation Center
Danbury Hospital Offsite, Outpatient Physical Therapy Center
235 Main Street
Danbury, CT 06810
(203) 730–5900; fax (203) 730–5905
Provides CDP/MLD by certified therapists.

Marietta B. Homberg, LMT
Washington Depot, CT
(860) 868–0794; fax (860) 868–0794
Certified CDP/MLD Therapist.

Delaware

Alfred I. duPont Hospital for Children
1600 Rockland Road
Wilmington, DE 19803
(302) 651–5600; fax (302) 651–5612
E-mail: webmaster@KidsHealth.org.
Website: http://KidsHealth.org/ai/service/lymphedema.html
Provides diagnosis and treatment of children with lymphedema.

Florida

Bayfront Medical Center Lymphedema Therapy Program
701 6th Street South
Saint Petersburg, FL 33701
(813) 893–6747 (phone and fax)
Provides CDP/MLD by certified therapists.

Baptist Outpatient Center
8950 North Kendall Drive
Miami, FL 33176
(305) 279–5188; fax (305) 273–2458
Provides CDP/MLD by certified therapists.

Blake Hospital Lymphedema Therapy Program
2020 59th Street West, 3 South
Bradenton, FL 34210
(941) 798–6190; fax (941) 798–6146
Provides CDP/MLD by certified therapists.

Gulf Coast Therapy Associates
3417A South Tamiami Trail
Port Charlotte, FL 33952
(941) 624–6222; fax (941) 624–6821
Provides CDP/MLD by certified therapists.

Halifax Medical Center
201 North Clyde Morris Boulevard, Suite 300
Daytona Beach, FL 32114
(904) 254–4001; fax (904) 947–4645
Provides CDP/MLD by certified therapists.

HealthQuest Complementary Therapy and Wellness Center
1526 Garden Street
Titusville, FL 32796
(407) 267–8141; fax (407) 267–7731
E-mail: li8ska@yourlink.net
Website: http://www.yourlink.net/li8ska
Provides CDP/MLD by certified therapists.

Koenig Natural Health
1400 Gulf Shore Boulevard
Naples, FL 34102

(941) 435–9921 (phone and fax)
Provides CDP/MLD by certified therapists.

Lerner Lymphedema Services, LC
Sawgrass Regional Medical Centre
12651 West Sunrise Boulevard
Sunrise, FL 33323
(800) 232–5542; fax (954) 845–9207
Provides CDP/MLD by certified therapists.

Lymphedema Institute of America, Inc.
PO Box 161889
Miami, FL 33116–1889
(800) 638–5843; fax (305) 265–0044
E-mail: RNLMT86@aol.com
Provides CDP/MLD by certified therapists.

Morton Plant Meese Healthcare
430 Pinellas Street
Clearwater, FL 33756
(813) 461–8179; fax (813) 461–8258
E-mail: masmldfl@msn.com
Provides CDP/MLD by certified therapists.

Mount Sinai Medical Center
4300 Alton Road
Miami Beach, FL 33140
(305) 674–2844; fax (305) 764–2038
Provides CDP/MLD by certified therapists.

Naples Community Hospital Outpatient Rehabilitation Center
302 Goodlette Road South
Naples, FL 34102
(941) 436–6712; fax (941) 436–6769
Provides CDP/MLD by certified therapists.

Nutrition and Health Center
300 Goodlette Road South
Grand Central Station
Naples, FL 34102

(941) 436–6755; fax (941) 436–6780
Provides CDP/MLD by certified therapists.

Wound Healing Lymphedema Center
5601 North Dixie Highway, Suite 107
Fort Lauderdale, FL 33334
(954) 772–8791; fax (954) 202–5611
E-mail: woundftl@aol.com
Provides comprehensive would healing and lymphedema therapy by trained
therapists, as well as lymphedema support groups.

Anthony Biviano, PT
4723 Northwest 30th Avenue
Gainesville, FL 32606
(352) 335–3687
Certified CDP/MLD therapist.

William Macdonald, LMT
P.O. Box 1697
Jensen Beach, FL 34958
(561) 334–0963
E-mail: bmacd@gatenet
Certified CDP/MLD therapist.

Edna R. Moore, LMT
125 Northeast 21st Street
Boca Raton, FL 33431
(561) 750–0622
Certified CDP/MLD therapist.

Ellen Gordon Poage, LMT
1650 Medical Lane, Suite 4
Fort Myers, FL 33907
(941) 939–1577; fax (941) 277–9289
E-mail: epoage@olsusa.com
Certified CDP/MLD therapist.

Veronika Snodgrass, LMT
3634 Lalani Boulevard
Sarasota, FL 34232

(941) 371–8684 (phone and fax)
Certified CDP/MLD therapist.

Margaret Tolman, RN
2200 North Atlantic Avenue
Daytona Beach, FL 32118
(904) 253–5095 (phone and fax)
Certified CDP/MLD therapist.

Georgia

Coliseum Medical Center
350 Hospital Drive, Building C
Macon, GA 31213
(912) 765–4884; fax (912) 765–4417
Provides CDP/MLD by certified therapists.

Compass Health Care
5671 Peachtree Dunwoody Road, Suite 560
Atlanta, GA 30342
(404) 252–9064; fax (404) 252–1541
Provides CDP/MLD by certified therapists.

Georgia Lymphedema Clinic
4122 East Ponce de Leon Avenue, Suite 10
Clarkstown, GA 30021
(404) 292–1754; fax (404) 296–2253
*Provides compression garments, skin care, pump therapy, and an exercise
program for lymphedema patients.*

HealthSouth Outpatient Center
3588 Riverside Drive
Macon, GA 31210
(912) 471–2140; fax (912) 471–2145
Provides CDP/MLD by certified therapists.

Memorial Medical Center Rehabilitation Department
4700 Waters Avenue
Savannah, GA 31404
(912) 350–7128; fax (912) 350–7131
Provides CDP/MLD by certified therapists.

Phoebe Physical Medicine Center
2336 Dawson Road, Suite 1100
Albany, GA 31707
(912) 888–8700; fax (912) 888–8715
Provides CDP/MLD by certified therapists.

Saint Joseph Hospital Rehabilitation Services
  Lymphedema Program
2260 Wrightsboro Road
Augusta, GA 30904
(706) 481–7359; fax (706) 481–7863
E-mail: casnkb@juno.com
Provides CDP/MLD by certified therapists.

Hawaii

Kapi'olani Women's Center
1907 South Beretania Street
Honolulu, HI 96826
(808) 973-5967; fax (808) 973-6537
Provides CDP/MLD by certified therapists.

Idaho

Idaho Elks Rehabilitation Hospital
204 Fort Place
Boise, ID 83702
(208) 333–2244; fax (208) 333–2309
Provides CDP/MLD by certified therapists.

Illinois

Evanston-Northwestern Healthcare Lymphedema Center
2650 Ridge Avenue
Evanston, IL 60201
(708) 570–2066; fax (847) 570–2901
Provides CDP/MLD by certified therapists.

Lake Forest Hospital Department of Rehabilitation Services
660 North Westmoreland Road
Lake Forest, IL 60045
(847) 234–6134; fax (847) 234–5646
Provides CDP/MLD by certified therapists.

Midwest Rehabilitation Services, Ltd.
40 South Clay Street, Suite 8W
Hinsdale, IL 60521
(630) 920–9204; fax (630) 920–9294
Provides CDP/MLD by certified therapists.

Rock Valley Physical Therapy
520 Valley View Drive
Moline, IL 61265
(309) 797–0866; fax (309) 797–0872
Provides CDP/MLD by certified therapists.

Saint Elizabeth's Hospital Outpatient Therapy
824 South 59th Street
Belleville, IL 62223
(618) 257–0366; fax (618) 234–9867
Provides CDP/MLD by certified therapists.

University of Illinois at Chicago Medical Center
1740 West Taylor
Chicago, IL 60612
(312) 996–3700; fax (312) 996–1457
Provides CDP/MLD by certified therapists.

Darek Zurawski, LMT
1147 Church Street
Northbrook, IL 60062
(847) 205–0211
Certified CDP/MLD therapist.

Indiana

Ball Memorial Hospital Rehabilitation Services
2401 University Avenue
Muncie, IN 47303
(765) 747–3239; fax (765) 741–1012
Provides CDP/MLD by certified therapists.

Daviess County Hospital Rehabilitation Services
1314 Grand Avenue
Washington, IN 47501
(812) 254–8889; fax (812) 254–8848
Provides CDP/MLD by certified therapists.

Healing Arts Center
1625 East Jefferson
Mishawaka, IN 46545
(219) 257–2200; fax (219) 257–2298
Provides CDP/MLD by certified therapists.

HealthSouth Tri-State Rehabilitation Hospital
4100 Covert Avenue
Evansville, IN 47714
(812) 476–9983; fax (812) 476–4270
Provides CDP/MLD by certified therapists.

Lutheran Hospital of Indiana Rehabilitation Services
7950 West Jefferson Boulevard
Ft. Wayne, IN 46804
(219) 435–7244; fax (219) 435–7628
Provides CDP/MLD by certified therapists.

Major Hospital Lymphedema Clinic
150 West Washington Street
Shelbyville, IN 46176
(317) 398–5300; fax (317) 392–6657
Provides CDP/MLD by certified therapists.

Methodist Hospital Lymphedema Therapy Program
Rehabilitation Center
303 East 89th Avenue
Merrillville, IN 46410
(219) 886–4617; fax (800) 839–6624
Provides CDP/MLD by certified therapists.

Saint Vincent Hospital Rehabilitation Services
2001 West 86th Street
Indianapolis, IN 46260
(317) 338–2269; fax (317) 338–2366
Provides CDP/MLD by certified therapists.

South Bend Memorial Hospital Lymphedema Therapy Program
615 North Michigan Street
South Bend, IN 46601
(888) 284–1068; fax (219) 284–1818
Provides CDP/MLD by certified therapists.

Frank Gentzke, LMT
6439 Hoover Road
Indianapolis, IN 46260
(317) 259–4983
Certified CDP/MLD therapist.

Iowa

Heartland Regional Resource Center
3047 Centerpoint Road NE
Cedar Rapids, IA 52402
(319) 297–7576; fax (319) 297–7587
Provides CDP/MLD by certified therapists.

Jaime Barker, LMT
Davenport, IA
(319) 322–0934
Certified CDP/MLD therapist.

Kansas

Therapy Concepts
12760 West 87th Street Parkway
Lenexa, KS 66215
(800) 227–1840 or (913) 438–8000; fax (913) 438–8008
E-mail: concepts@qni.com or info@therapyconcepts.com
Websites: http://www.therapyconcepts.com
              http://www.lymphology.com
*Provides CDP/MLD by certified therapists. Therapy Concepts was the first
outpatient clinic in the United States to get Medicare coverage for lymphedema therapy.*

Via Christi Regional Medical Center
1151 North Rock Road
Wichita, KS 67206
(316) 634–3495; fax (316) 634–1141
Provides CDP/MLD by certified therapists.

Kentucky

Baptist Hospital East
4000 Kresge Way

Louisville, KY 40207
(502) 897–8137; fax (502) 896–7259
Provides CDP/MLD by certified therapists.

Central Baptist Hospital Rehabilitation Services
1740 Nicholasville Road
Lexington, KY 40503
(606) 275–6144; fax (606) 275–6430
Provides CDP/MLD by certified therapists.

Louisiana

HealthSouth Rehabilitation Hospital of Baton Rouge
8595 United Plaza Boulevard
Baton Rouge, LA 70809
(504) 927–0567; fax (504) 926–2357
Provides CDP/MLD by certified therapists.

Louisiana Physical Therapy Centers, Inc.
1305 Texas Avenue
Alexandria, LA 71301
(318) 443–5278; fax (318) 443–1906
Provides CDP/MLD by certified therapists.

Carrie Ann Wiedemann, LMT
3017 12th Street
Metairie, LA 70002
(504) 455–6462; fax (504) 838–0156
E-mail: clareese@doulton.com
Certified CDP/MLD therapist.

Maine

Betty Jane St. Jean-Lomas, LMT
161 Main Street
Lubec, ME 04652
(207) 733–2567
Certified CDP/MLD Therapist.

Maryland

Johns Hopkins Hospital
Physical Medicine and Rehabilitation Department
600 North Wolfe Street
Baltimore, MD 21287–5189
(410) 614–3234; fax (410) 614–2065
Provides CDP/MLD by certified therapists.

Mid-Atlantic Lymphedema Center
600 Ridgely Avenue, Suite 230
Annapolis, MD 21401
(800) 845–7525; fax (410) 997–0001
Provides CDP/MLD by certified therapists.

Mid-Atlantic Lymphedema Center
1131 Baltimore Pike
Bel Air, MD 21014
(800) 845–7525; fax (410) 997–0001
Provides CDP/MLD by certified therapists.

Mid-Atlantic Lymphedema Center
5010 Dorsey Hall Drive
Ellicott City, MD 21042
(800) 845–7525; fax (410) 997–0001
Provides CDP/MLD by certified therapists.

Mid-Atlantic Lymphedema Center
11119 Rockville Pike
Rockville, MD 20852
(800) 845–7525; fax (410) 997–0001
Andrea Delamura, PT, Certified CDP/MLD Therapist
Provides CDP/MLD by certified therapists.

Pamela Sabatiuk, OT
1356 Splashing Brook Court
Eldersburg, MD 21784
(410) 795–7507
E-mail: SSteinb673@aol.com
Certified CDP/MLD therapist

James Salander, MD
11119 Rockville Pike
Rockville, MD 20852
(301) 881–5503; fax (301) 468–3609
Vascular surgeon who diagnoses and treats lymphedema.

Massachusetts

Acupuncture & Associated Therapies
Deer Crossing, Upper Level
Mashpee, MA 02649
(508) 539–0299
Provides CDP/MLD by certified therapists.

Baystate Medical Center Physical Therapy Department
759 Chestnut Street
Springfield, MA 01199
(413) 784-4279; fax (413) 784-8525
Provides CDP/MLD by certified therapists.

Fallon Clinic
135 Goldstar Boulevard
Worcester, MA 01610
(508) 856–9510; fax (508) 853–1907
Provides CDP/MLD by certified therapists.

Lahey Clinic Lymphedema Treatment Clinic
41 Mall Road
Burlington, MA 01805
(781) 273–5100; fax (781) 744-2832
Provides CDP/MLD by certified therapists.

Lerner Lymphedema Services
1 Hawthorne Place, Suite 103
Boston, MA 02114
(617) 367–6162; fax (617) 367–6114
Provides CDP/MLD by certified therapists, as well as training for certified CDP/MLD therapists.

Janice Hebert, LMT
131 Main Street
Lancaster, MA 01561

(978) 368–0696 or (978) 368–0663
E-mail: mldmona@aol.com
Certified CDP/MLD therapist.

Heather McElroy, LMT
129 Stafford Street
Charlton, MA 01507
(508) 2480–6612; fax (508) 248–5282
E-mail: Heather@binaryheaven.com
Certified CDP/MLD therapist.

Michigan

Annette's Boutique
3646 Rochester Road
Troy, MI 48083
(248) 680–1600; fax (248) 680–2174
Provides CDP/MLD by certified therapists.

Beaumont Rehabilitation and Health Center
746 Purdy
Birmingham, MI 48009
(248) 258–3700; fax (248) 258–0685
Provides CDP/MLD by certified therapists.

Henry Ford Hospital
2799 West Grand Boulevard
Detroit, MI 48202
(313) 876–1245; fax (313) 876–2930
Provides CDP/MLD by certified therapists.

Henry Ford Wyandotte Hospital Outpatient Clinic
3200 Biddle, Third Floor
Wyandotte, MI 48192
(734) 284–4499; fax (734) 284–4696
Provides CDP/MLD by certified therapists.

Karmanos Cancer Institute Lymphedema Management Program
4100 John R.
Detroit, MI 48201

(313) 745–4645; fax (313) 993–0307
Provides CDP/MLD by certified therapists, as well as classes in self care and support groups.

Mary Free Bed Outpatient Therapy Center
350 Lafayette Southeast
Grand Rapids, MI 49503
(616) 242–9250; fax (616) 242–0085
Provides CDP/MLD by certified therapists.

Michigan Lymphedema Clinic
2900 Hannah Boulevard, Suite B102
East Lansing, MI 48823
(517) 336–4559; fax (517) 332–3961
Provides CDP/MLD by certified therapists.

Munson Medical Center
Munson Community Health Center
1105 6th Street
Traverse City, MI 49684
(616) 935–8600; fax (616) 935–8609
Provides CDP/MLD by certified therapists.

Saint Joseph Mercy Hospital Rehabilitation Services
5301 East Huron River Drive
Ann Arbor, MI 48106
(734) 712–4926; fax (734) 712–3532
Provides CDP/MLD by certified therapists.

Sparrow Hospital Lymphedema Program
2900 Hannah Boulevard, Suite B102
East Lansing, MI 48823
(517) 336–4570; fax (517) 332–3961
Provides CDP/MLD by certified therapists.

Barbara Starke, RN
508 Pleasant Street
Saint Joseph, MI 49085
(616) 983–4990; fax (616) 849–1470
Certified CDP/MLD Therapist.

Minnesota

Abbott Northwestern Hospital
Sister Kenney Institute
Lymphedema Therapy Program
800 East 28th Street
Minneapolis, MN 55407–3799
(612) 863–4446; fax (612) 863–5698
Provides CDP/MLD by certified therapists.

Fairview University Medical Center Rehabilitation Services
420 Delaware Street SE
Minneapolis, MN 55455
(612) 626–8400; fax (612) 626–1118
Provides CDP/MLD by certified therapists.

Mayo Clinic Lymphedema Clinic
200 First Street SW
Rochester, MN 55905
(507) 266–8913; fax (507) 266–1561
Provides CDP/MLD by certified therapists.

Jean Finley, OT
2903 Edgerton Street
Little Canada, MN 55117
(612) 490–1874
Certified CDP/MLD tdherapist.

Mohammad Noori, LMT
8224 Oxborough Avenue
Bloomington, MN 55437
(612) 831–8681; pager 3195911
Certified CDP/MLD therapist.

Irene Waldridge, LMT
1074 Legion Street
Shakopee, MN 55379
(612) 445–7578
E-mail: bobwld@pclink.com
Certified CDP/MLD therapist

Missouri

HealthSouth Lymphedema Therapy Program
955 Executive Parkway
St. Louis, MO 63141
(314) 469–5454; fax (314) 469–8728
Provides CDP/MLD by certified therapists.

Physicians Services, LLC
522 North New Ballas, Suite 280
St. Louis, MO 63141
(314) 692–7700; fax (314) 692–0440
Provides CDP/MLD by certified therapists.

Northeast Regional Medical Center Lymphedema Clinic
Patterson Campus
PO Box C8502
Kirksville, MO 63501–8599
(888) 785–7770 or (660) 785–3747; fax (660) 785–3723
Provides CDP/MLD by certified therapists.

Regional Center for Sports Medicine and Rehabilitation
Cox Medical Plaza I, Suite 300
Springfield, MO 65807
(800) 790–3980 or (417) 269–5500; fax (417) 269–5508
Provides CDP/MLD by certified therapists.

Virginia L. Melnick, LMT
3237 Patrick Lane
Pacific, MO 63069
(314) 271–2428
Certified CDP/MLD therapist who offers education about prevention and treatment of lymphedema, as well as pain management.

Nebraska

Fremont Area Medical Center
450 East 23rd Street
Fremont, NE 68025
(402) 727–3329; fax (402) 727–3339
Provides CDP/MLD by certified therapists.

Nebraska Methodist Hospital Rehabilition Partners
8303 Dodge Street
Omaha, NE 68114
(402) 354–4670; fax (402) 354–3226
Provides CDP/MLD by certified therapists.

Nevada

HealthSouth Rehabilitation Hospital of Reno
Lymphedema Therapy Program
555 Gould at Mill Street
Reno, NV 89502
(702) 348–5566; fax (702) 348–5610
Provides CDP/MLD by certified therapists.

New Hampshire

Sportsworks/Optima Healthcare
1 Highlander Way
Manchester, NH 03104
(603) 625–2131; fax (603) 625–2213
Provides CDP/MLD by certified therapists.

New Jersey

Clara Maass Medical Center
Rehabilitation Services
1 Clara Maass Drive
Belleville, NJ 07109
(973) 450–2050; fax (201) 844–4939
Provides CDP/MLD by certified therapists.

Healthsouth Outpatient Rehabilitation Hospital of Tom's River
Lymphedema Therapy Program
1451 Route 37 West
Tom's River, NJ 08755
(732) 818–3600; fax (732) 341–0252
Provides CDP/MLD by certified therapists.

Heartland Rehabilitation Services
2630 East Chestnut Avenue
Vineland, NJ 08361

(609) 692–1483; fax (609) 692–7423
Provides CDP/MLD by certified therapists.

Lymphedema Therapy, Inc.
14 Beechwood Road
Basking Ridge, NJ 07920
(908) 696–0200; fax (908) 696–0211
E-mail: lti@bellatlantic.net
Provides CDP/MLD by certified therapists.

Mid-Atlantic Lymphedema Center
52 Forest Avenue
Paramus, NJ 07652
(800) 660–1608; fax (201) 587–8520
Provides CDP/MLD by certified therapists.

Mountainside Hospital
Department of Physical Rehabilitation
Bay and Highland Avenues
Montclair, NJ 07042
(973) 429–6050; fax (973) 680–7917
Provides CDP/MLD by certified therapists.

Rumson Therapeutic & Sports Massage Center
16 West River Road
Rumson, NJ 07760
(201) 450–2050
Provides CDP/MLD by certified therapists.

Saint Barnabas Medical Center Physical Therapy Department
Old Short Hills Road
Livingston, NJ 07039
(973) 533–8990; fax (973) 533–8305
Provides CDP/MLD by certified therapists.

Somerset Medical Center Physical Therapy Department
110 Rehill Avenue
Somerville, NJ 08876
(908) 685–2944; fax (908) 685–2531
Provides CDP/MLD by certified therapists.

Marlene Cuniberti, LMT
42 Hillside Avenue
Englewood, NJ 07631
(201) 569–8731 (phone and fax)
E-mail: easthill@compuserve.com
Certified CDP/MLD therapist.

Donna DiPoce, DC
1899 Monitor Drive
Toms River, NJ 08753
(732) 506–9654; fax (732) 929–2756
Certified CDP/MLD therapist who provides education and referrals for lymphedema patients.

Roseanna Ellis, LMT
823 Locust Street
Roselle Park, NJ 07204
(908) 245–9124
Certified CDP/MLD therapist who provides treatment, education, and referrals.

Phillip Kilcoyne, LMT
146 West Upper Ferry Road
West Trenton, NJ 08628
(609) 882–9595
Certified CDP/MLD therapist.

Guenter Klose, LMT
27G Chicopee Drive
Princeton, NJ 08540–1715
(609) 924–9615; fax (609) 924–9623
E-mail: guenter@sprintnet.com
Certified CDP/MLD therapist and instructor.

Leslie Walker, OT
2630 East Chestnut Avenue
Vineland, NJ 08361
(609) 692–1483
Certified CDP/MLD therapist.

New Mexico

HealthSouth Rehabilitation Hospital
7000 Jefferson NE
Albuquerque, NM 87109
(505) 344–9478; fax (505) 345–6772
Provides CDP/MLD by certified therapists.

Marie Smeriglio, LMT
Santa Fe, NM
(505) 986–0237; fax (505) 954–4310
E-mail: maries@mci.2000.com
Certified CDP/MLD therapist.

New York

Creséra Wellness Center
471 Willis Avenue
Williston Park, NY 11596
(516) 747–1382; fax (516) 747–1507
E-mail: jfklymph@li.net
Provides CDP/MLD by certified therapists.

Delmar Physical Therapy Associates and Lymphedema
    Treatment Center
8 Booth Road
Delmar, NY 12054
(518) 439–1485; fax (518) 478–0850
Provides CDP/MLD by certified therapists.

Energy Works
14 West 55th Street, #4B
New York, NY 10019
(212) 459–9705
Provides CDP/MLD by certified therapists.

Glens Falls Hospital Lymphedema Therapy Program
102 Park Street
Glens Falls, NY 12801
(518) 761–5333; fax (518) 761–2416
Provides CDP/MLD by certified therapists.

Helen Hayes Hospital Lymphedema Therapy Program
Route 9W
West Haverstraw, NY 10993
(914) 786–4358
Provides CDP/MLD by certified therapists.

Holbrook Wellness Center
5000 Expressway Drive South
Holbrook, NY 11741
(516) 588–0149; fax (516) 585–7575
Provides CDP/MLD by certified therapists.

Hudson Valley Physical Therapy and Lymphedema Services
PO Box 705
Larchmont, NY 10538
(914) 946–5409; fax (914) 946–5409, star 51
E-mail: blobel@erols.com
Provides CDP/MLD by certified therapists.

J.T. Mather Memorial Hospital
Lymphedema Treatment Center
75 North Country Road
Port Jefferson, NY 11777
(516) 476–2737; fax (516) 476–2791
Provides CDP/MLD by certified therapists.

Jin Shin Do
15 Parkway
Katohah, NY 10536
(914) 225–9590 (phone and fax)
Provides CDP/MLD by certified therapists.

Lerner Lymphedema Services
245 East 63rd Street, Suite 106
New York, NY 10021
(800) 848–1015 or (212) 688–6107; fax (212) 688–6159
E-mail: Lymphdoc@bridge.net
Website: http://www.lymphedemaservices.com
*Patient treatment center and headquarters for the largest school in the
United States for training therapists and physicians in CDP/MLD
throughout the United States.*

Lourdes Hospital
169 Riverside Drive
Binghamton, NY 13905
(607) 798–5255; fax (607) 798–5192
Provides CDP/MLD by certified therapists.

Lymphedema Management Center of Western New York
3768 Seneca Street
West Seneca, NY 14224
(716) 674–7780; fax (716) 674–7781
E-mail: kjt-scg@att.net
Provides CDP/MLD by certified therapists.

Lymphedema Therapy Treatment Center
77 Froehlich Farm Boulevard
Woodbury, NY 11797
(800) MD–LYMPH or (516) 364–2200; fax (516) 364–1844
Provides a broad spectrum of diagnostic and treatment modalities for lymphedema patients.

Memorial Sloan-Kettering Cancer Center Lymphedema
    Therapy Program
1275 York Avenue
New York, NY 10021
(212) 639–7833; fax (212) 794–6237
Provides CDP/MLD by certified therapists and physiatrists.

Nu-Tech Comprehensive Lymphedema Services, Ltd.
3180 Expressway Drive South
Islandia, NY 11722
(800) 698–2192; fax (516) 234–2205
Provides CDP/MLD by certified therapists.

Southampton Hospital Breast Health Center
Physical Therapy Rehabilitation Department
Lymphedema Therapy Program
240 Meeting House Lane
Southampton, NY 11988
(516) 726–1468; fax (516) 726–8483
Provides CDP/MLD by certified therapists.

United Health Services Hospitals
Wilson Memorial Regional Medical Center
Department of Medical Rehabilitation
33-57 Harrison Street
Johnson City, NY 13760
(607) 763–5200; fax (607) 763–6853
Provides CDP/MLD by certified therapists.

University Hospital and Medical Center—Stony Brook
Department of Physical and Occupational Therapy
Lymphedema Therapy Program
33 Research Way
East Setauket, NY 11733
(516) 444–4240; fax (516) 444–4713
Provides CDP/MLD by certified therapists.

Westbury Total Health Care
265 Post Avenue, Suite 100
Westbury, NY 11590
(516) 333–3253 or (516) 536–4931; fax (516) 333–8452
Provides manual lymphatic drainage and instruction in self-care for lymphedema patients.

Polly Correa Jiacovelli, LMT
1270 Fifth Avenue, Apartment 9B
New York, NY 10029
(212) 369–7536
Certified CDP/MLD therapist.

Robin Landau, LMT
664 East Beech Street
Long Beach, NY 11561
(516) 432–4113; fax (516) 432–4616
Certified CDP/MLD therapist.

Elizabeth Marcari, LMT
522 Old Stone Highway
East Hampton, NY 11937
(516) 267–6957
Certified CDP/MLD therapist.

Zinaida Pelkey, DO
180 West 80th Street
New York, NY 10024
(212) 787–2884; fax (212) 787–3954
Certified CDP/MLD therapist.

Deborah S. Sarnoff, MD
Cosmetique
31 Northern Boulevard
Greenvale, NY 11548
(516) 484–9000; fax (516) 484–7549
Dermatologist and laser surgeon experienced in treating the skin problems of lymphedema patients.

Deborah S. Sarnoff, MD
625 Park Avenue
New York, NY 10021
(212) 794–4000; fax (212) 794–0231
Dermatologist and laser surgeon experienced in treating the skin problems of lymphedema patients.

Annie Siegel, LMT
45 West 95th Street
New York, NY 10025
(212) 961–0355
Certified CDP/MLD therapist.

Jim Slaymaker, LMT
Huntington, NY
(516) 652–7533
Certified CDP/MLD therapist.

North Carolina

Charlotte Institute of Rehabilitation Lymphedema
   Management Program
1100 Blythe Boulevard
Charlotte, NC 28203
(704) 355–4465; fax (704) 355–7873
Provides CDP/MLD by certified therapists.

East Carolina University Department of Physical Therapy
Belk Building
Greenville, NC 27858–4353
(919) 328–4449; fax (919) 328–0707
Provides CDP/MLD by certified therapists.

Moses Cone Outpatient Rehabilitation Center
1904 North Church Street
Greensboro, NC 27405
(910) 271–4840; fax (910) 271–4921
Provides CDP/MLD by certified therapists.

Ultimate Health Center, Inc.
31 College Place
Asheville, NC 28801
(800) 268–6905
Provides CDP/MLD by certified therapists.

Ultimate Health Center, Inc.
2097 North Fork Right Fork Road
Black Mountain, NC 287110
(704) 669–1053; fax (704) 669–1047
E-mail: uhc@primeline.com
Website: http://members.xoom.com/uhc/
Provides CDP/MLD by certified therapists.

James Tracy, PT
Greenville, NC
(919) 321–8275
Certified CDP/MLD therapist.

North Dakota

Physical Therapy and Occupational Therapy Associates
550 13th Avenue East
West Fargo, ND 58078
(701) 282–0011; fax (701) 282–0022
Provides CDP/MLD by certified therapists.

Ohio

Mount Carmel East Hospital
6001 East Broad Street
Columbus, OH 43213
(614) 234–6464; fax (614) 234–6720
Provides CDP/MLD by certified therapists.

Mount Carmel East Hospital Women's Health Center
5965 East Broad Street
Columbus, OH 43213
(614) 234–8100
Provides CDP/MLD by certified therapists.

Mount Sinai Center for Breast Health
26900 Cedar Road, Suite 310
Beachwood, OH 44122
(216) 595–2600; fax (216) 595–2578
Provides CDP/MLD by certified therapists.

Tri-State Lymphedema Clinic
7565 Kenwood Road, Suite 203
Cincinnati, OH 45236
(513) 793–7710; fax (513) 793–2770
E-mail: lymph@one.net
Website: http://lymph.com/frmain.htm
Offers evaluation, education, consultation, treatment, and support for pa-tients with lymphedema or edema associated with various other conditions.

University Hospital of Cleveland Lymphedema Center
11100 Euclid Avenue
Cleveland, OH 44106
(216) 844–7868; fax (216) 844–8964
Provides CDP/MLD by certified therapists.

Donna Barkett, LMT
5035 Mayfield Road, Suite 209
Lyndhurst, OH 44124
(216) 291–3305
Certified CDP/MLD therapist.

Howard Douglas, LMT
PO Box 861
Chesterland, OH 44026
(216) 729–3258; fax (216) 729–2648
Certified CDP/MLD therapist.

Kathryn Sample, RN
P.O. Box 74
Morrow, OH 45152
(513) 877-2559; voice mail (513) 877-2600; fax (513) 877-2558
E-mail: Kgsample@aol.com
Certified CDP/MLD therapist.

Oklahoma

Hillcrest Medical Center
Lymphedema Clinic
1826 East 15th Street, Suite B
Tulsa, OK 74119–1122
(918) 749–2252 or (918) 579–7163; fax (918) 579–7110
Provides CDP/MLD by certified therapists.

NovaCare Outpatient Rehabilitation
3700 North Classen Boulevard, Suite 200
Oklahoma City, OK 73118
(800) 745–7463 or (405) 528–0500; fax (405) 528–0522
E-mail: edemaland1@aol.com
Provides CDP/MLD by certified therapists.

Oregon

Acupressure Health Care
215 Southeast 6th Street, Suite 307
Grants Pass, OR 97526
(541) 479–9481
Provides CDP/MLD by certified therapists.

Legacy Good Samaritan Hospital
Cancer Rehabilitation
1015 Northwest 22nd Avenue
Portland, OR 97210

(503) 413–7283; fax (503) 413–6920
Provides CDP/MLD by certified therapists.

Whole Body Therapy
530 NW 3rd Street, Suite A
Newport, OR 97365
(541) 265–8680
Provides CDP/MLD by certified therapists.

Pennsylvania

Body Therapy Center and School of Body Therapies
931 Langhorne-Yardley Road
Langhorne, PA 19047-1368
(215) 752–7666; fax (215) 752–1909
Provides CDP/MLD by certified therapists.

Breast Cancer Physical Therapy Center
Recovery in Motion Rehabilitation Program
1905 Spruce Street
Philadelphia, PA 19103
(215) 772–0160; fax (215) 772–0342
Provides CDP/MLD by certified therapists.

Chestnut Hill Rehabilitation Hospital
8601 Stenton Avenue
Wyndmoor, PA 19038
(215) 233–6240; fax (215) 233–6234
Provides CDP/MLD by certified therapists.

D.T. Watson Rehabilitation Hospital Lymphedema
    Therapy Program
301 Camp Meeting Road
Sewickley, PA 15143
(800) 922–4226; fax (423) 539–6797
Provides CDP/MLD by certified therapists.

Dynamic Rehabilitation Services
8080 Old York Road, Suite 204
Elkins Park, PA 19027

(215) 782–8760; fax (215) 635–7130
Provides CDP/MLD by certified therapists.

Fox Chase Cancer Center Lymphedema Therapy Program
7701 Burholme Avenue
Philadelphia, PA 19111
(215) 728–2592; fax (215) 728–3873
Provides CDP/MLD by certified therapists.

Genesis Eldercare Rehabilitation Services
148 West State Street
Kennett Square, PA 19348
(800) 220–3123; fax (610) 279–8360
Provides CDP/MLD by certified therapists.

Good Shepherd Rehabilitation Hospital
501 St. John's Street
Allentown, PA 18103
(610) 776–3220; fax (610) 776–3551
Provides CDP/MLD by certified therapists.

Guthrie Health Care Systems Lymphedema Clinic
Guthrie Square
Sayre, PA 18840
(717) 882–4801; fax (717) 882–5830
Provides CDP/MLD by certified therapists.

John Heinz Institute of Rehabilitation Medicine
Outpatient Clinic
150 Mundy Street
Wilkes-Barre Township, PA 18702
(717) 830–2020; fax (717) 830–2027
Provides CDP/MLD by certified therapists.

Lymphatic Care Specialists, LLC
285 Parker Road
Eatontown, PA 07724
(732) 923–9300
Provides CDP/MLD by certified therapists.

Lymphedema Relief Center
218 Center Road

Monroeville, PA 15146
(412) 829–7608; fax (412) 374–1416
Provides CDP/MLD by certified therapists.

Magee Women's Hospital Physical Therapy Department
300 Halket Street
Pittsburgh, PA 15213
(412) 641–4480; fax (412) 641–1093
Provides CDP/MLD by certified therapists.

Mid-Atlantic Lymphedema Center
9150 Marshal Street
Philadelphia, PA 19114
(800) 677–7179; fax (610) 328–5205
Provides CDP/MLD by certified therapists.

Mid-Atlantic Lymphedema Center
631 South Chester Road
Swarthmore, PA 19081
(800) 677–7179; fax (610) 328–5205
Provides CDP/MLD by certified therapists.

MossRehab Outpatient Center
100 Old York Road
Jenkintown, PA 19046
(215) 884–9050; fax (215) 884–1713
Provides CDP/MLD by certified therapists.

Penn State Geisinger Rehabilitation Hospital Lymphedema
   Treatment Center
GHP Lane
Danville, PA 17822-2414
(717) 271–6594; fax (717) 271–5852
Provides CDP/MLD by certified therapists.

The Lymphedema Connection PC
Webster Hall, Suite 145
4415 Fifth Avenue
Pittsburgh, PA 15213
(412) 682–6335; fax (412) 682–6352
E-mail: TLCPC15213@aol.com
Provides CDP/MLD by certified therapists.

Therapeutic Rehabilitation and Athletic Care
5100 Peach Street
Erie, PA 16509
(814) 864–5097; fax (814) 864–9583
Provides CDP/MLD by certified therapists.

Mary Pat House, RN
Monroeville/Pittsburgh, PA
(412) 829–7608 or (412) 829–3037
Certified CDP/MLD Therapist.

Jane Kepics, PT
Eagleville, PA
(610) 539-5732
Certified CDP/MLD therapist.

Wilma Morgan, OT
Collegeville, PA
(610) 489–9535
Certified CDP/MLD therapist.

Rhode Island

Directions in Healing
528 North Main Street, 4th Floor, Suite 3
Providence, RI 02904
(401) 272–8584; fax (401) 421–4037
Provides education, consultations, and referrals.

Ellen Belconis, LMT
482 Roundhill Court
Warwick, RI 02886
(401) 781–8155
Massage therapist who provides education, information, and referrals.

South Carolina

McLeod Regional Medical Center
Rehabilitative Services
555 East Cheves Street

Florence, SC 29501
(864) 667–2043; fax (864) 667–2051
Provides CDP/MLD by certified therapists.

South Dakota

Sioux Valley Hospital Outpatient Rehabilitation Center
3401 West 49th Street
Sioux Falls, SD 57106
(605) 333–1860; fax (605) 333–1857
Provides CDP/MLD by certified therapists.

Nancy Everist, LMT
225 East 28th Street
Sioux Falls, SD 57105
(605) 336–6962
Certified CDP/MLD therapist.

Tennessee

Baptist Memorial Hospital Women's Health Center
6025 Walnut Grove Road, Suite 101
East Memphis, TN 38120
(901) 226–0590; fax (901) 226–5563
Provides CDP/MLD by certified therapists.

Complementary and Integrative Medicine Group
105 Donner Road
Oak Ridge, TN 37831
(423) 482–0981; voice mail (423) 927–1701; fax (423) 482–0959
Provides CDP/MLD by certified therapists.

HealthSouth Chattanooga Rehabilitation Hospital
2412 McCallie Avenue
Chattanooga, TN 37404
(423) 697–9133; fax (423) 697–9295
Provides CDP/MLD by certified therapists.

Saint Thomas Hospital
4220 Harding Road
Nashville, TN 37205

(615) 222–6671 or (615) 222–5553; fax (615) 222–6345
Provides CDP/MLD by certified therapists.

The Therapy Center West
8904 Cross Park Drive
Knoxville, TN 37923
(423) 690–2671; fax (423) 690–6445
E-mail: scmoozey@aol.com
Provides CDP/MLD by certified therapists.

Wellmont Holston Valley Medical Center
130 West Ravine Street
Kingsport, TN 37660
(423) 224–5510; fax (423) 224–5568
Provides CDP/MLD by certified therapists.

Teri Craig, LMT
3614 Wilbur Place
Nashville, TN 37204
(615) 385–4600
Certified CDP/MLD therapist.

Connie Davis, RN
20208 Crowne Brook Circle
Franklin, TN 37067
(615) 771-7784
Certified CDP/MLD therapist.

Texas

All Saints Hospital Rehabilitation Services Lymphedema Center
1400 8th Avenue
Fort Worth, TX 76104
(817) 922–2530; fax (817) 922–2534
Provides CDP/MLD by certified therapists.

Canapa MLD Services
3112 Highlawn Terrace
Fort Worth, TX 76133
(817) 346–2036 or (817) 346–0983
E-mail: acanapa@startext.net
Provides CDP/MLD by certified therapists.

Edema and Wound Care Clinic
8200 Wednesbury Lane, Suite 110
Houston, TX 77074
(800) 624–7196
Provides CDP/MLD by certified therapists.

HealthSouth
Lymphedema Therapy Program
17506 Red Oak Drive
Houston, TX 77070
(281) 580–1212; fax (281) 580–7827
Provides CDP/MLD by certified therapists.

HealthSouth Rehabilitation Hospital
Lymphedema Therapy Program
515 West 12th Street
Texarkana, TX 75501
(903) 793–0088; fax (903) 793–0899
Provides CDP/MLD by certified therapists.

Lymphedema and Wound Care Clinic of Austin
5750 Balcones Drive, Suite 110
Austin, TX 78731
(512) 453–1930; fax (512) 467–6851
Provides CDP/MLD by certified therapists.

Lymphedema Services of Texas
5282 Medical Drive, Suite 170
San Antonio, TX 78229
(800) 435–5512; fax (210) 616–0927
Website: http://www.lymphedemarx.com/drw/guide.html
Provides CDP/MLD by certified therapists.

Rio Vista Rehabilitation Hospital
1740 Curie Drive
El Paso, TX 79902
(915) 543–6966; fax (915) 532–5587
Provides CDP/MLD by certified therapists.

Ida Gaither, LMT
3851 Meadowdale Lane
Dallas, TX 75229

(214) 902–0214
Certified CDP/MLD therapist.

Barbro Hesselager, LMT
14500 San Pedro, Suite 205
San Antonio, TX 78232
(210) 545–6062; fax (210) 342–4707
E-mail: barling@texas.net
Certified CDP/MLD therapist.

Maggie Williams, PT
Houston, TX
(281) 556–6129
Certified CDP/MLD therapist.

Martha Zenger, LMT
5747 Birdwood Road
Houston, TX 77096–2108
(713) 776–8533 (phone and fax)
Certified CDP/MLD therapist and instructor.

Utah

Intermountain Health Care Lymphedema Therapy Program
34 East 600 South
St. George, UT 84770
(435) 634–4545; fax (435) 634–4519
E-mail: Igm@infowest.com
Provides CDP/MLD by certified therapists.

University of Utah Hospitals and Clinic Rehabilitation Services
Lymphedema Therapy Program
50 North Medical Drive
Salt Lake City, UT 84108
(801) 581–2619; fax (801) 585–3060
Provides CDP/MLD by certified therapists.

Utah Valley Regional Medical Center
1034 North, 500 West
Provo, UT 84604
(801) 357–7540; fax (801) 357–7725
Provides CDP/MLD by certified therapists.

Vermont

Timberlane Physical Therapy
40 Timber Lane
South Burlington, VT 05403
(802) 864–3785; fax (802) 864–0274
E-mail: leslipt@vbimail.champlain.edu
Provides CDP/MLD by certified therapists.

Virginia

Halcyon Therapies
10405 Gordon Road
Spotsylvania, VA 22553
(540) 785–1678
Provides CDP/MLD by certified therapists.

Lymphodynamics
1168 First Colonial Road, Suite 5
Virginia Beach, VA 23454
(757) 481–7985; fax (757) 481–4638
Provides CDP/MLD by certified therapists.

Massey Cancer Center
Cancer Rehabilitation Program
1300 East Marshall
Richmond, VA 23298
(804) 828–9901; fax (804) 828–9857
Provides CDP/MLD by certified therapists.

Tidewater Physical Therapy
12420 Warwick Boulevard, Suite 6K
Newport News, VA 23606
(757) 599–5551; fax (757) 595–5238
Provides CDP/MLD by certified therapists.

John Guarino, LMT
3313 Wyndham Circle, #4209
Alexandria, VA 22302
(703) 671–7790
Certified CDP/MLD therapist and instructor.

Homer Scott, LMT
Newport News, VA
(804) 642–6675
Certified CDP/MLD therapist.

Washington

Anne Warjone Healing Massage
2200 24th Avenue East
Seattle, WA 98112
(206) 328–0910; voice mail (206) 320–1032; fax (206) 328–2310
Provides CDP/MLD by certified therapists.

Lake Union Massage & Healing Touch
1818 Westlake Avenue North
Seattle, WA 98109
(206) 282–0172
Provides manual lymph drainage, as well as instruction in managing lymphedema and preventing flare-ups.

Lymphatic Therapy Associates
1800 Northwest Market, Suite 206
Seattle, WA 98107
(206) 784–6988; fax 206-782-2079
E-Mail: lymphclinic@seanet.com
Provides CDP/MLD by certified therapists.

Saint Luke's Rehabilitation Institute
Lymphedema Services
711 South Cowley
Spokane, WA 99201
(800) 982–6141; fax (509) 458–6117
Provides CDP/MLD by certified therapists.

West Virginia

HealthSouth Mountainview Regional Rehabilitation Hospital
1160 Van Voorhis Road
Morgantown, WV 26505
(304) 598–1100; fax (304) 598–1103
Provides CDP/MLD by certified therapists.

Wisconsin

Dean Therapy Center
1806 West Beltline Highway
Madison, WI 53713
(608) 250–1485
Provides CDP/MLD by certified therapists.

Dean Therapy/Princeton
1726 Eagan Road
Madison, WI 53704
(608) 246–2644
Provides CDP/MLD by certified therapists.

Canada

Caring Hands Massage Clinic
1095 Whitefield Drive
Peterborough, ON K9J 7P4
(705) 748–0771 (phone and fax)
Provides CDP/MLD by certified therapists.

Hunt Club Physiotherapy Clinic
204-2446 Bank Street
Ottawa, Ontario K1V 1A4
(613) 247–1245; fax (613) 247–1246
E-mail: hcphysio@cyberus.ca
Website: http://www.worldsites.net\hcphysio
Provides CDP/MLD by certified therapists.

Osmose Center
2225 Autoroute-Des
Laval, Quebec H7S 126
(514) 688–1144
Provides CDP/MLD by certified therapists.

Robert Harris, LMT
PO Box 5701
Victoria, BC V8R 6S8
(250) 598–9862 (phone and fax)
Certified CDP/MLD therapist and instructor.

Internet/WWW Help

Elana Hayden
Creative Research Company
Division of *Creative Graphic Design*
(718) 264–0724; fax (718) 454–1722
E-mail: hayden@bway.net
Website: http://www.creativegraphicdesign.com
Assistance in computer use and accessing on-line services.

Other

Joyce Hart
12 Woodhill Drive
Redwood City, CA 94061
(650) 366–4278; fax: (650) 364–8687
Motivational speaker who provides counseling, education, and referrals for people with primary and secondary lymphedema.

RESEARCH PROJECTS

Lymphedema Family Study
University of Pittsburgh Department of Human Genetics
A300 Crabtree Hall, GSPH
Pittsburgh, PA 15261
(412) 624–4657; fax (412) 624–3020
Website: http://www.pitt.edu/~genetics/lymph/lymph.htm
This is a clinical genetic research study of people with primary lymphedema which is supported by a grant from the D.T. Watson Rehabilitation Hospital in Sewickley, PA. The study accepts families with two or more individuals who have lymphedema.

Molecular Genetics Study of Lymphedema
Mansoor Sarfarazi, PhD
Surgical Research Center
Department of Surgery
University of Connecticut Health Center
263 Farmington Avenue
Farmington, CT 06030–1110
(860) 679–3629 (office); (860) 679–3923 (laboratory);
    fax (860) 679–7524 or (860) 679–2451
E-mail: msarfara@cortex.uchc.edu

A study of families in which lymphedema appears that aims to identify a specific small region of a chromosome shared by most if not all affected individuals. The study involves both affected and unaffected members of families with different forms of lymphedema.

Marlys Witte, MD, and Charles Witte, MD
University of Arizona Health Sciences Center Department
    of Surgery
1501 North Campbell Avenue
PO Box 245063
Tucson, AZ 85724-5063
(510) 626–6118; fax (520) 626–0822
E-mail: lymph@u.arizona.edu
A multifaceted research project that includes study of lymphatic and blood-vessel formation, genes that are involved in familial lymphedema syndromes, the biology and pathobiology of lymphatic tissues, lymphatic-system imaging, and therapeutic approaches to enhancing or reducing the proliferation of lymphatic and blood vessels.

SCHOOLS

Academy of Lymphatic Studies
10753 US HWY #1
Sebastian, FL 32958
(800) 863-8935; fax (561) 589-0306
Website: www.acols.com or www.acols.net

The largest school in the U.S. that offers comprehensive courses and certification in lymphedema therapy. Courses are given at Lerner Lymphedema Services centers and other locations throughout the country.

Casley-Smith Training Program—Australia
Judith Casley Smith, PhD
c/o Henry Thomas Laboratory
University of Adelaide
SA 5005, Australia
61+(8) 8271–2198; fax 61+(8) 8271–8776
Email: casley@enternet.com.au
Offers training in manual lymph drainage and complete decongestive physiotherapy.

Dr. Vodder School—Austria
Alleestrasse 30, A-6344
Walschsee, Tyrol
Austria
011–43–5374–5245 (Austria); (212) 737–6203 (U.S.);
   fax 011–43–5374–5245–4
Offers complete certification program in Dr. Vodder's manual lymph drainage and combined decongestive therapy for the treatment of lymphedema.

Dr. Vodder School—North America
PO Box 5701
Victoria, BC V8R 6S8, Canada
(250) 598–9862 (phone and fax)
E-mail: drvodderna@vodderschool.com
Website: http://www.vodderschool.com/
Offers complete certification program in Dr. Vodder's manual lymph drainage and combined decongestive therapy for the treatment of lymphedema.

International Academy of Lymphology
PO Box 1954
Orem, UT 84059
(800) 975–0123; fax (801) 224–1545
E-mail: ial@ial.org
Website: http://www.ial.org
Provides home-study program for professionals and lay people that teaches the causes and prevention of lymphedema through six two-hour video tapes, four audiotapes, and the textbook "The Golden Seven Plus One." The IAL has certified 1,000 lymphologists worldwide and publishes a bi-yearly journal, "Lymphology."

Privatschule Földi
Zurn Engelberg 18
79249 Merzhausen, Germany
011 497 6140 6921; fax 011 497 6140 6983

SUPPORT GROUPS

The following is a list of telephone numbers to contact lymphedema support groups by geographic area. Please telephone the groups directly for information about meeting places and times.

Alaska

Anchorage: (907) 243–8360
Wasilla: (907) 376–3037

Arizona

Mesa: (602) 830-4756
Phoenix: (602) 235-9130 or (602) 837–0191
Tucson: (800) 34–LYMPH
Tucson: (520) 742–5661

California

Concord: (510) 674–2125
Monterey: (408) 394–4196 or (408) 645–4570
Newport Beach: (714) 760–5645
Orange: (714) 731–0233
Palm Springs (619) 251–9686 or (760) 251–9686
Sacramento (916) 729–2889 or (916) 422–5973
San Diego: (760) 434–3599
San Jose: (888) GINGERK or (408) 445–8626; fax (408) 723–3797
Santa Barbara: (805) 682–7111
Santa Clarita: (805) 254–2763

Colorado

Colorado Springs: (719) 599–8457
Denver: (303) 973–8618

Connecticut

Danbury: (203) 790–6568 or (203) 744–3586 (upper limb lymphedema only)
Stamford: (203) 378–2297 or (203) 325–1544
Waterbury: (203) 758–6138

Florida

Fort Lauderdale: (954) 772–8791
Fort Myers: (941) 454–1810
Jacksonville: (904) 745–6800
Miami: (305) 595–3999
Miami (Spanish-speaking group): (305) 598–9233
Naples: (941) 514–3845, fax (941) 514–3846 (breast-cancer-related lymphedema only)

Orlando: (407) 897–6701
Zephyrhills: (813) 783–6123

Georgia

Albany: (912) 888–8700
Atlanta (greater Atlanta area): (770) 442–1317

Hawaii

Koloa, Kauai: (808) 742–1840

Illinois

Glenn Ellyn: (630) 790–3264
Northbrook: (847) 498–1255

Indiana

Fort Wayne: (219) 637–3069
Mishawaka: (219) 257–2200

Kansas

Overland: (800) 227–1840

Louisiana

Baton Rouge: (504) 924–8450

Massachusetts

Boston (greater Boston area): (718) 894–2309

Maryland

Ellicott City: (800) 845–7525 or (410) 964–4400
North Bethesda (Rockville): (301) 881–5503

Michigan

Northern Michigan: (616) 228–6359

Minnesota

Minneapolis: (612) 626–5913
St. Paul: (612) 432–0014

New York

Brooklyn: (718) 965–3160
Buffalo/Elma: (716) 652–9383
Ghent: (518) 392–2151
Garden City: (800) 877–8077
Guilderland: (518) 452–3456
Hauppauge: (516) 757–8899
Kingston: (914) 336–5402
Rochester: (716) 234–1290
Southampton: (516) 726–2111
Stony Brook: (516) 444–4240

New Jersey

Princeton: (201) 673–3714 or (732) 495–3915
Sewell: (609) 589–3955

North Carolina

Charlotte: (704) 355–1502
Greensboro: (336) 299–1456

Ohio

Columbus: (614) 876–5976
Cleveland: (216) 844–7868

Oklahoma

Oklahoma City: (405) 840–1829

Oregon

Pendleton: (541) 938–3208

Pennsylvania

Monroeville: (412) 829–7608
Pittsburgh: (412) 899–3312
Sewickley: (800) 922–4226 or (412) 749–2289

Rhode Island

Providence: (401) 454–0404

South Dakota

Sioux Falls: (605) 333–5244

Tennessee

Cleveland: (423) 476–8319
Knoxville: (800) 225–8129

Texas

Houston: (713) 723–4174

Virginia

Northern Virginia: (703) 909–0299
Virginia Beach/Norfolk: (757) 481–7985

Washington

Seattle: (206) 782–5598
Walla Walla: (541) 938–3208

Wyoming

Rawlins: (307) 328–1809

Canada

Toronto, Ontario: (416) 533–2428

Recommended Reading

LYMPHEDEMA

Dinclaux, Arlette J. *Nutritherapy for Lymphedema.* Desert Hot Springs, CA: E.S.O.P. Publishing, 1995.

Wittlinger, Hildegard, Guenther Wittlinger, and Ingrid Kurz. *Textbook of Dr. Vodder's Manual Lymph Drainage,* 5th ed. Portland, OR: Medicina Biologica, 1995.

CANCER

Batt, Sharon. *Patient No More: The Politics of Breast Cancer.* Charlottetown, P.E.I., Canada: Gynergy Books, 1994.

Diamond, W. John, and W. Lee Cowden, with Burton Goldberg. *An Alternative Medicine Definitive Guide to Cancer.* Tiburon, CA: Future Medicine Publishing, Inc., 1997.

Kradjian, Robert M. *Save Your Life from Breast Cancer.* New York: Berkley Publishing, 1994.

Moss, Ralph. *Cancer Therapy, The Independent Consumer's Guide to Non-Toxic Treatment and Prevention.* New York: Equinox Press, 1995.

Phillips, Robert H. *Coping with Prostate Cancer.* Garden City Park, NY: Avery Publishing Group, 1994.

Swirsky, Joan, and Barbara Balaban. *The Breast Cancer Handbook: Taking Control After You've Found a Lump,* rev. ed. Staten Island, NY: Power Publications, 1998.

Walters, Richard. *Options: The Alternative Cancer Therapy Book.* Garden City Park, New York: Avery Publishing Group, 1993.

GENERAL MEDICAL INFORMATION

Baldwin, Fred D., and Suzanne McInerney. *Infomedicine: A Consumer's Guide to the Latest Medical Research.* New York: Little Brown & Co., 1996.

Complete Drug Reference. Yonkers, NY: Consumer Reports Books, 1998.

Public Citizen Health Research Group. *Health Letter.* Monthly newsletter. Public Citizen Health Research Group, 1600 20th Street NW, Washington, DC 10009; (202) 588–1000.

ALTERNATIVE MEDICINE

Achterberg, Jeanne. *Imagery in Healing.* Boston: New Science Library, Shambhala, 1985.

Alternative Health and Medicine Encyclopedia, 2nd ed. Detroit: Gale Research Inc., 1997.

Alternatives for the Health Conscious Individual. Monthly newsletter. Mountain Home Publishing, 2700 Cummings Lane, Kerriville, TX 78028; (210) 367–4492.

Balch, James F., and Phyllis A. Balch. *Prescription for Nutritional Healing,* 2nd ed. Garden City Park: Avery Publishing Group, 1997.

Beinfield, Harriett, and Efrem Korngold. *Between Heaven and Earth: A Guide to Chinese Medicine.* New York: Ballantine Books, 1991.

Benson, Herbert. *The Relaxation Response.* New York: Outlet Books, 1993.

Chopra, Deepak. *Quantum Healing.* New York: Bantam Books, 1989.

Cummings, Stephen, and Dana Ullman. *Everybody's Guide to Homeopathic Medicine.* Los Angeles: J.P. Tarcher, Inc., 1991.

Elman, Dave. *Hypnotherapy.* Glendale, CA: Westwood Publishing Co., 1984.

Feldman, John, ed. *Hands On Healing.* Emmaus, PA: Rodale Press, 1989.

Fine, Donald I. *Transcendental Meditation*. New York: Roth Robert, 1998.

Goleman, Daniel, and Joel Gurin, eds. *Mind-Body Medicine: How to Use Your Mind for Better Health*. Yonkers, NY: Consumer Reports Books, 1993.

Janiger, Oscar, and Philip Goldberg. *A Different Kind of Healing*. New York: Putnam Books, 1993.

Weil, Andrew. *Health and Healing*. Boston: Houghton Mifflin Company, 1988.

Williams, Wendy. *The Power Within*. New York: HarperCollins, 1990.

DIET AND NUTRITION

Deskins, Barbara, and Jean E. Anderson. *The Nutrition Bible: The Comprehensive, No-Nonsense Guide to Foods, Nutrients, Additives, Preservatives, Pollutants and Everything Else We Eat and Drink*. New York: William Morrow & Co., 1997.

Kirschmann, Gayla J., and John D. Kirschmann. *Nutrition Almanac*, 4th ed. New York: McGraw-Hill, 1996.

Larson, Roberta Duyff. *The American Dietetic Association's Complete Food & Nutrition Guide*. Minnetonka, MN: Chronimed Publishing, 1996.

Kushi, Michio. *The Macrobiotic Way: The Complete Macrobiotic Diet & Exercise Book*. Garden City Park, NY: Avery Publishing Group, 1993.

National Women's Health Network. *The Diet Your Doctor Won't Give You*. Washington, DC: National Women's Health Network, 1987.

Spear, Ruth. *Low Fat and Loving It*. New York: Warner Books, 1991.

Stepaniak, Joanne. *Uncheese Cookbook: Creating Amazing Dairy-Free Cheese Substitutes*. Summertown, TN: Book Publishing Company, 1994.

Tierra, Lesley. *The Herbs of Life*. Freedom, CA: Crossing Press, 1992.

Woodruff, Sandra. *Secrets of Living Fat-Free*. Garden City Park, NY: Avery Publishing Group, 1997.

Zukin, Jane. *Dairy-Free Cookbook*. Rocklin, CA: Prima Books, 1991.

SELF-HELP

McCue, Kathleen. *How To Help Children Through A Parent's Serious Illness*. New York: St. Martin's Press, 1996.

White, Barbara J., and Edward J. Madara, eds. *The Self-Help Sourcebook: Finding & Forming Mutual Aid Self-Help Groups*. Denville, NJ: Self-Help Clearing House, 1995.

Stutz, David, and Bernard Feder. *The Savvy Patient: How to Be an Active Participant in Your Medical Care*. Yonkers, NY: Consumer Reports Books, 1990.

Index

BC Cancer Agency
Vancouver - Library
Vancouver, BC Canada

BC Cancer Agency
Vancouver - Library
675 West 10th Ave.
Vancouver, BC Canada
V5Z 1L3